Praise for *Anxiety D*

"A wonderfully practical handbook with straightforward illustrations drawn from experience to inform sensible and systematic application of therapeutic concepts to everyday practice."

Lee Wang, M.D.
Psychiatrist, Michigan State University
East Lansing, Michigan

"Dr. van Ingen's holistic, evidence-based approach to anxiety is inspiring. Packed with multiple specific, concrete, and accessible examples, this book is a helpful resource for practitioners and clients alike."

Stacy Freiheit, Ph.D.
Clinical Psychologist
Associate Professor, Augsburg College
Minneapolis, Minnesota

"Cleverly thoughtful and chock-full of easy-to-read and practical advice, Dr. van Ingen has successfully given both clinicians and consumers valuable tools and insights to address one of the mental health fields most common and challenging psychiatric disorders—Anxiety. The book ("Anxiety Disorders Made Simple: Treatment Approaches to Overcome Fear and Build Resiliency") makes a laudable contribution to the application and treatment of anxiety disorders by extracting often heavily theoretical ideas and perspectives, and translating them into meaningful and common-sense clinical strategies and techniques. With a robust array of clinical examples and pertinent vignettes that skillfully illustrate a wide-spectrum of anxiety-based disorders, Dr. van Ingen has proven himself to be not only a sophisticated clinician, but also an inspiring teacher. His book has a fresh approach that is delightfully "laser beam" in its focus and execution. Above all, it offers a wealth of practicality and wisdom that makes it a "must-read" for anyone interested in dealing with the challenges of anxiety and its complex manifestations."

James M. Riggio, Ph.D.
Staff Psychologist
John D. Dingell VA Medical Center
Detroit, Michigan

"Dr. van Ingen has nailed it! He effectively combined scientist-practitioner and lay understandings of core concepts related to assessment & intervention in a friendly read for providers and consumers alike. From the very first pages, including a beautifully written acknowledgements section and relevant review of the literature, through the final paragraphs, including resources for providers and consumers, *Anxiety Disorders Made Simple* is a must have for the professional clinician's library. As a clinician, I learned a lot by reading this book. I am encouraged knowing Dr. van Ingen's unique style of articulating evidence based practices will help the masses manage their anxiety via this publication, a highly complex, evidence based resource made simple. As an educator in general, I applaud Dr. van Ingen's use of clear syntax as well as prose that are illuminated by captivating analogies and case examples."

Jameson C. Lontz, Ph.D.
Executive Director, Blue Mountain
Neuropsychological Associates
Assistant Professor of Counselor Education &
Master of Counseling Program Director
Gonzaga University
Spokane, WA

"Dr. van Ingen's book, *"Anxiety Disorders Made Simple: Treatment Approaches to Overcome Fear and Build Resiliency"* is of great value to any clinician who practices, or who wants to practice, Cognitive Behavioral psychotherapy. Evidence-based treatment is an essential component of the contemporary practice of psychotherapy, and Dr. van Ingen presents both the theory and clinical application of Cognitive Behavioral psychotherapy, which has an impressive track record in the treatment of psychiatric disorders. Anxiety reduction, given its widespread prevalence in clinical settings, is a component of all treatment plans. Whether you are a psychotherapist who wants to incorporate elements of this approach into your treatment repertoire, or are developing the skills to become a Cognitive Behavioral psychotherapist this book is essential reading."

Alan F. Dubro, Ph.D.
Clinical Psychologist
Tarrytown, New York

"Anxiety Disorders Made Simple is a comprehensive guide to treating anxiety that includes all of the top cognitive-behavioral anxiety management strategies as well as valuable information about the therapeutic relationship, diet, and exercise. Adeptly directed toward clinicians, Daniel van Ingen, PsyD. supports his work with neuroscience and research while still delivering his promise to keep it simple. Dr. van Ingen provides dozens of useful proven strategies with his own creative twists and original ideas based on his clinical experience. He artfully utilizes metaphors, thoughtful quotes, and case examples to effectively illustrate his ideas and keep the reader engaged. The table of contents makes this a great reference guide to easily access his techniques."

Jennifer L. Abel, Ph.D. author of
Active Relaxation and
Resistant Anxiety, Worry, and Panic: 86 Practical
Treatment Strategies for Clinicians.

"Superbly edited and written......Its depth and breadth are impressive. This book is particularly well suited for professionals in mental health. A must read book by practitioners who want to learn evidence-based approaches for treating anxiety disorders."

Magn Nyang, Ed.D.
Clinic Director
Minnesota Multicultural Counseling and consultant Inc.
Author of *Acculturation of Ethiopian and Somali Immigrant*
Adolescents: Acculturation Orientation of Immigrant
Youths in the United States

"I am impressed, inspired and invigorated by reading *Anxiety Disorders made Simple.* I appreciate the clearly delineated interventions and the ease with which you discuss differences and similarities among anxiety problems. I feel your writing and your explanations cultivate approaching clients from a strengths perspective which also captures your amazing healing spirit. Bravo on your synthesis of interventions from interoceptive exposure to mindfulness and the value of acceptance. Your rich synthesis of interventions is clinical treasure."

Kileen Smyth, MSW, LICSW
Mayo Clinic Department of Psychiatry & Psychology
Rochester, Minnesota

"Dr. van Ingen has combined his expertise and experience to create a concise and user-friendly toolkit. As a psychologist specializing in anxiety disorders, I am thrilled to have a new and insightful resource, chock full of both traditional and cutting-edge ideas and wisdom. Dr. van Ingen's willingness to share his knowledge with fellow therapists is inspiring."

Patricia H. Price, PsyD
Psychologist, Private Practice
Rochester, Minnesota

Anxiety Disorders Made Simple

Treatment Approaches to Overcome Fear and Build Resiliency

by

DANIEL J. VAN INGEN, PSYD

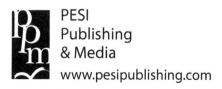

PESI
Publishing
& Media
www.pesipublishing.com

For the sake of confidentiality, numerous details concerning names, descriptions, geographical locations, and other aspects of the case vignettes in this work have been altered by the author. However, these alterations of the details have been done in a way that has preserved the treatment dynamics disclosed in the examples.

Published by
PESI Publishing & Media
PESI, Inc
3839 White Ave
Eau Claire, WI 54703

Printed in the United States of America

ISBN: 978-1-936128-97-6

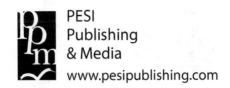

PESI
Publishing
& Media
www.pesipublishing.com

This book is dedicated to all of my loving family, with boundless gratitude.
To my wife, Sarah, my best friend. You are the love of my life.
To my parents: Your love and support endure through victories and setbacks.
To my sisters: You are fearless mothers and strong women.
To my children—Majestic, Blaze, and Freedom: May you always be unafraid to leave your comfort zone, willing to challenge your fears head on with courage and resilience, and be willing to take the steps in life to lift your vision higher.

Table of Contents

Acknowledgments

There are many people I would like to acknowledge as this book emerges as a mental health resource. But, my deepest appreciation is for my wife, Sarah–you demonstrated tremendous resilience over the last few years in obtaining your Ph.D. You have inspired me on the value of harnessing anxiety in the pursuit of a goal. When we were pushed close to the breaking point, you still found ways to encourage and challenge me. I appreciate your kindness, warmth, and unwavering love. And, I appreciate your willingness to embrace hardship for long-term gain. Now, as a professor, you are developing your evidence-based research program aimed to help bridge research and practice. Your passion has helped this book project emerge from the ebb and flow of discouragement toward hopefulness and influence others from the lab to the clinic.

I want to thank my father, John van Ingen, Ph.D., University of St. Thomas, whose philosophy teaching with Machiavelli, Hobbes, Nietzsche, Descartes, and Kant continues to challenge and educate college students. You encouraged me to "enjoy the excitement and power of ideas and learn to defend the ones worth defending" which impacted the development of this book. I would like to thank Christopher Vye, Ph.D., Advisor and Chair of the University of St. Thomas Graduate School of Professional Psychology. Your commitment to specific factors and treatment outcome research has influenced me toward the golden mean–balancing common factors in my psychotherapy work with evidence based treatment methods, critical for the treatment of anxiety. I want to express appreciation to John Buri, Ph.D., a former advisor whose "Learning and Memory" course at the University of St. Thomas in St. Paul, Minnesota establishes a foundation for future clinicians on negative reinforcement and anxiety treatment. I am thankful for our many talks on vignettes and life principles that started over 20 years ago.

I would like to thank my mentor Dave Novicki, Ph.D., an anxiety expert at Michigan State University. Your nuggets of wisdom are memorable and long-lasting, with a few being incorporated as quotes in this book. I am grateful to a colleague in the Psychology Department at Augsburg College in Minneapolis, Minneapolis, Stacy Freiheit, Ph.D., who has collaborated with me on research studies, including our meta-analysis on effectiveness studies of cognitive behavioral therapy for anxiety disorders. I would like to thank Alan Dubro, Ph.D., a New York psychologist, whose expertise in psychological assessment and diagnostic differentiation has enriched my clinical skills. I have appreciated your perspective on many case consultations.

I would like to thank my editor, Marietta Whittlesey, who has provided outstanding input. I want to thank you for your clinical perspective, the invaluable formatting and editorial assistance you provided to this project. I am also thankful to Claire Zelasko, Linda Jackson, Michael Olson, Marnie Sullivan, Karsyn Morse, Shannon Becker, and the many others at PESI and CMI Education Institute Inc.

The contents of this book are based upon the research, wisdom, and theoretical conceptualization written about by numerous colleagues who have spent their professional lives studying professional psychology, anxiety treatment, and cognitive-behavioral therapy. Many colleagues have shown dedication and commitment to improving the quality of life for individuals with anxiety. I am grateful to many colleagues for these psychological breakthroughs. In particular, I want to thank Aaron T. Beck, M.D., father of cognitive therapy, University of Pennsylvania. You have been a pioneer in the development of cognitive-behavioral therapy. In addition, I would like to thank the following (although this by no means entails a complete listing): Dean McKay, Ph.D., Fordham University; Martin Seligman, Ph.D., University of Pennsylvania; Judith Beck, Beck Institute for Cognitive Behavior Therapy and University of Pennsylvania; Jonathan Abramowitz, Ph.D., University of North Carolina; David Tolin, Ph.D., Anxiety Disorders Center at Institute of Living; Edna Foa, Ph.D., University of Pennsylvania School of Medicine; Robert DeRubeis, Ph.D., University of Pennsylvania; David Barlow, Ph.D., University of Vermont; Steven Hollon, Ph.D., Vanderbilt University; Patricia Resick, Ph.D., Boston University; Martin Antony, Ph.D., Ryerson University.

I would also like to thank those many other individuals who helped in the development of this book. Von Sheppard, my college counselor who experientially taught me the positive impact of counseling, and my first college friend Rene Rodriguez, who continually challenged me to leave my comfort zone. I want to thank Kileen Smyth, Clinical Social Worker and Therapist at Mayo Clinic, whose long walks and talks on the south campus of the University of St. Thomas 20 years ago was influential for me on mindfulness, non-judgment, and compassion for others. I am grateful to my best man Bill Rademacher, whose wise counsel over the years has been a consistent pillar in my life. And, I want to emphasize that you have been an advocate for the idea that even one visit can be life-changing for somebody.

There are many others who have contributed to this book. I am grateful to the many colleagues from Cohort 13 at the University of St. Thomas Graduate School of Professional Psychology. I am grateful to Jim Riggio, Ph.D. at the John D. Dingell VA Medical Center in Detroit, Michigan. I appreciate Linda Moore and my other colleagues and behavioral intervention experts at Chrestomathy, Inc., Minneapolis, Minnesota. I am thankful to Training Director Tawa Sina, Ph.D. particularly for cultural formulation training, past supervisors Decolius Johnson, Ph.D., and Jen Grzegorek, Ph.D., as well as my colleagues, in particular, Lee Wang, M.D., and the 2007 Intern class from the Michigan State University Counseling Center. Last, but most importantly, I want to thank the One who has said so often "Do Not Be Afraid."

About the Author

Daniel van Ingen, Psy.D., is a Licensed Psychologist in Michigan, Minnesota, and Florida. He received his BA degree from the University of St. Thomas, his MA degree from Saint Mary's University, and his Doctor of Psychology (Psy.D.) from the University of St. Thomas Graduate School of Professional Psychology. His research interests include anxiety treatment, parenting research, and intellectual disabilities. Clinically, Dr. van Ingen specializes in anxiety and trauma-based disorders in southwest Florida and manages a private practice called Anxiety Shrinks! He is a national speaker and has presented research at national and international conferences for over 10 years. He blogs anxiety articles and posts weekly parenting podcasts on his website www.danvaningen.com. Dr. van Ingen and his wife Dr. Sarah van Ingen have three children and live in Sarasota, Florida.

Introduction

Most of the techniques presented in this book are based on clinical research. I have tried to maintain and honor the complexity of the critical concepts taken from clinical research and the key cognitive behavioral therapy tenets. At the same time, I've avoided the jargon that often enters into the scholarly discipline of psychology. Many counselors, therapists, social workers, and psychologists do not review research literature and incorporate the ideas into their practice. There are many factors that contribute to the gap between research and practice. Sometimes this gap is due to a lack of time on the part of practitioners, and sometimes this is due to dissemination issues, among other factors. In many cases, the fact that clients typically seen in outpatient clinics and private practices are often more complex than those selected to participate in randomized clinical trials (RCT's) contributes to the gap (Spinazzola, Blaustein, & van der Kolk, 2005). The emergence of effectiveness research that emphasizes external validity designed to supplement RCT's is an attempt to bridge the research to practice gap (Stewart & Chambless, 2009; van Ingen & Novicki, 2009; van Ingen, Freiheit, & Vye, 2009).

By design, the practical applications of effectiveness research findings are more apparent to practitioners than the applications of RCT findings. The way effectiveness studies are written makes it easier for clinicians to understand how the interventions would work in a practice setting, because clients with multiple problems are included and treatment flexibility is incorporated into the studies. This book is also an attempt to help bridge the gap between research and practice for clinicians.

In chapter 1, the major features of each of the primary anxiety disorders are discussed as "core patterns." Tables for each of the anxiety disorders are provided with the core patterns, a typical psychological goal for each pattern, and a matching intervention for each of the core patterns. Case examples are provided throughout this chapter as strategies to address the central problems of each anxiety disorder.

Chapter 2 transitions from differences between anxiety disorders to similarities among anxiety problems. Effective intervention requires accurate interpretations during the clinical assessment to achieve diagnostic differentiation. However, the identification of common features of anxiety problems, such as fear of anxiety and external locus of control, is central to the goal of this chapter. A "Laser Beam" intervention is identified for each of the 10 common anxiety features emphasized in this chapter.

Chapter 3 focuses on trauma therapy. Two types of trauma, small and big, are identified in this chapter. Human unresolved responses to trauma (HURTS)—self-centeredness, insecurity resulting from attachment problems, inconsistency in relationships, cynicism, and disagreeableness—are articulated. The chapter includes 20 remedies for 20 PTSD DSM-5® symptoms. Additional topics that are discussed include mindfulness, a combination of remedies for dissociation problems, and positive psychology interventions that supplement trauma therapy.

Chapter 4 is written for those therapists wanting to get more out of and give more to anxious clients. This chapter separates those clients ready for challenging treatment versus those clients who need supportive therapy. Many clients with anxiety disorders need relationship building, professional counseling, and basic problem-solving. For those clients ready for the "big leagues," this chapter will build emotional muscle that can increase anxiety tolerance. Included are the challenges of interoceptive exposure (producing uncomfortable sensations in session to increase tolerance), the ramifications of medication therapy, clarity on what negatively reinforces anxiety, and experimental actions that initially raise anxiety but reframe exaggerated beliefs.

Chapter 5 emphasizes the heart of cognitive therapy – the core belief. The pertinent issues of psychotherapy research and recent debates on what works in treatment are elaborated. Core beliefs are categorized: (1) defective – effective, (2) degree of responsibility, (3) control – freedom, and (4) trust – safety. The treatment of these belief categories are aptly illustrated using cognitive, behavioral, and experiential strategies.

Working with trauma survivors is a major source of stress, and sometimes even vicariously traumatic. Treating anxiety entails swimming through lots of emotion and difficulty. It can be intricately grueling. At the same time, the work can be deeply satisfying. Chapter 6 provides guidance on the "Big 3" for clients with anxiety: good sleep hygiene, regular exercise, and good nutrition. Chapter 6 is intended to conceptualize this "Big 3" as a critical component in treatment delivery. It is also important for helping therapists to stay balanced and healthy.

CHAPTER 1

Freedom from Fear

Each of the Anxiety Disorders has Core Patterns

Decades of research on anxiety have provided clarity on the central features of each of the anxiety disorders. In chapter 1, these features are identified as "core patterns." These core patterns are consistent with the symptom criteria in the *Diagnostic and Statistical Manual of Mental Disorders, 5th edition* (DSM-5®, American Psychiatric Association (APA), 2013). When therapists hear about a problem, establishing a goal and identifying an intervention within a therapeutic relationship is routine standard practice. The objective in this chapter is to name matching interventions for each of the core patterns while providing case examples.

Goal of Evidence-Based Psychological Treatment

I have worked side by side with numerous behavior analysts, professional counselors, nurses, social workers, and psychologists. Being a treatment provider requires a ton of work and lots of struggles. I've been a seminar speaker for over 10 years in a variety of contexts. When I ask the audience the tough question, "has anyone lost a patient due to suicide?" the number of hands raised often surprises me. The honesty that is communicated in a mental health field that inherently promotes narcissism is inspiring. Recently, at seminars in New Jersey and Wisconsin, the majority of people raised their hands.

Dealing with all facets of suicide is one of the dreaded tasks of a therapist. Professionals with extensive experience will say that they can deal with these decisions methodically and proficiently. The work life of a therapist is very difficult at times. It is full of ups and downs and often involves hands getting dirty.

Another challenge is finding ways to apply the right treatments to complicated problems. The goal of evidence-based psychological treatment for

1

anxiety disorders is to help patients become less afraid. While this may involve being less anxious in social situations for those with social anxiety, lots of anxiety treatment involves having less fear of anxiety itself. One of the terms cognitive-behavioral therapists use in a variety of research and clinical contexts is "anxiety tolerance." This basically means becoming more comfortable with anxiety.

Sometimes headaches limit work and relationship functioning. Most of us endure the day even if we have a headache. "Oh, I have a headache, but I'll be all right." The headache may limit a strength workout or a 5-mile jog, but we tend to move along in life. Similarly, "Oh, I'm experiencing some panic feelings but I'll be all right." For a person being treated for an anxiety disorder, coming to a place of tolerance of the anxiety is a standard treatment goal. When I work with people, my goal is to bring them to a place of having freedom from fear and anxiety.

F.E.A.R.: FALSE EVIDENCE THAT APPEARS REAL

F.E.A.R. is false evidence that appears real. My goal for anyone who comes into my office is to have freedom from the fears that can control their lives. Anxiety is not fear, precisely, because fear involves an objective danger like the mugger a man faces in the alley. Instead, anxiety is a kind of fear that is imagined and perceived (real versus imagined danger). Fear comes from real danger that is definite and immediate. In contrast, anxiety is not the result of something specific, but comes from one's vision of possible dangers, chronic worries, and continuous what if's. These emotional states are interrelated and they influence each other. These emotional states cause attention to narrow, limiting a client's ability to process information (Easterbrook, 1959). Clients tend to have a selective attentional bias for threat during emotional arousal (Barlow, 2002). This is why the false evidence appears real–everything is being perceived through a limited and narrow lens.

> *If we wish to conquer undesirable emotional tendencies in ourselves, we must … cold-bloodedly go through the outward motions of those contrary dispositions we prefer to cultivate.*
>
> William James

This book is written in a straight-forward manner with an interest in sharing the tools that have helped others gain control over their lives, learn to tolerate their anxiety, and gain freedom from and mastery over their fears. It is written for clinicians who help clients gain freedom from fear and anxiety and strengthen their sense of being unafraid of fear.

ASSESSMENT VERSUS INTERVENTION

When clients come in for appointments, the standard goal for therapists is to collaboratively work to discover the presenting problems. One of the psychology fundamentals providers learn in their Ph.D. programs or professional psychology graduate schools is the difference between assessment and intervention. Assessment is related to understanding the problem. Intervention is related to solutions for the problems. Sometimes psychology consumers notice that they can soak in a lot of good information from a self-help book. Psychology is great at providing information or understanding of a particular problem, but you may have noticed that psychology can sometimes offer very little in terms of solutions to problems.

> *Ignorance is bliss. Not knowing something is often more comfortable than knowing it.*
>
> E. D. Hirsch, Jr.

It is not uncommon for educated college students to figure out their own diagnoses by their own reading and the utilization of on-line screening tools. Of course, they understand the caveats, but many college counselors know that these educated consumers are not way off in their hypotheses.

The issue is that assessment (or diagnosis) may be about acquiring information, but intervention requires something unique that is most often obtained from an experienced therapist. While assessment involves understanding the problem, intervention is related to the solution to the problem.

The primary assessment activity is a diagnostic evaluation, sometimes referred to as an initial assessment (IA). Subsequent to assessment, therapists sometimes engage in psychoeducation. It is important that psychoeducation not be confused with treatment. When therapists provide a handout on sleep hygiene, or provide education on concentration differences in mania versus ADHD, or normalize nightmare activity following trauma, these are psychoeducation activities. Psychoeducation involves information about the diagnosis or psychological problem, an expression of understanding that helps destigmatize, and provision of a rationale for relevant treatment modalities.

In contrast, intervention is related to treatment. When clinicians reframe one of the most common cognitive errors, emotional reasoning, or do an exposure treatment, these are intervention activities. For clients experiencing fears and having problems being hampered by anxiety, this book is intended to highlight the key intervention activities providers can use to bring about insight that helps clients experience clarity on their misperceptions.

THE ASSESSMENT OF CORE PATTERNS IN ANXIETY

Accurate assessment is critical for freedom from fear and anxiety. There are many overlapping symptoms among anxiety disorders. And, there are key differences. Below are the core patterns within the primary anxiety disorders. The core patterns of panic disorder are anxiety sensitivity, persistent worry about panicking, and chronic fear of bodily sensations. The core patterns of generalized anxiety disorder (GAD) are uncontrollable worry, future orientation, negative cognitive biases, somatic arousal, role and task inefficiency, and interpersonal aversiveness that includes avoidance. The core patterns of social phobia are self-focused attention, negative self-evaluation, anxious apprehension, social avoidance and escape, and skills deficits.

> *There is a time when we must firmly choose the course we will follow, or the relentless drift of events will make the decision for us.*
>
> Herbert V. Prochnow

The core patterns in obsessive-compulsive disorder (OCD) are obsessions–unwanted, repeated, intrusive thoughts, images, or urges that result in significant anxiety, e.g., contamination, religious, sexual or aggression–and compulsions or behaviors designed to reduce anxiety–checking, washing, counting or repeating. The core patterns of post-traumatic stress disorder (PTSD) include the major clusters of re-experiencing, avoidance, numbing, and hyperarousal symptoms as well as fears of memories, depression, guilt and survival guilt, reduction in awareness of surroundings, derealization, and depersonalization.

CORE PATTERN INTERVENTIONS IN ANXIETY

For core anxiety problems, there are a variety of solutions that center on becoming unafraid of fear and anxiety. The goal of anxiety interventions is to reduce fear and help increase emotional muscle, or anxiety tolerance.

When I lived in Minnesota, I once worked with a woman named Lisa who had panic disorder. Lisa was a 25-year old college student working at a supermarket chain paying her way through college. Lisa's father was authoritarian and very demanding. Once, when Lisa was helping her parents host some guests, she drove over from her apartment for the dinner. During the meal, she helped some of the guests with coffee. Rather than bring the pot to the dinner table, she brought a guest's mug to the counter. Lisa's father stood up and shouted at her about bringing the pot to the table. Lisa ran downstairs and had a panic attack.

UNAFRAID OF PANIC

Lisa met criteria for panic disorder and had a persistent concern about future panic attacks. Her anxiety escalated around her father and when she was in uncomfortable situations like having more than two customers in her cashier line at the supermarket. Her processing of internal cues often triggered her panic, and the panic felt like it came out of nowhere. Whenever she experienced a physical symptom, like

> A single event can awaken within us a stranger totally unknown to us.
>
> Antoine de Saint-Exupery

shortness of breath, her perception was one of tunnel vision, and she focused like a laser beam on her bodily sensations. She then magnified her symptoms, and other symptoms occurred like chest pressure, heart palpitations, and dizziness. This led to catastrophic misinterpretations of her symptoms and escalating symptoms of panic.

Panic is tolerable. The essential goal of panic treatment is anxiety tolerance. Accordingly, we began to practice cognitive reappraisals of the panic attack symptoms in different ways. Progress for Lisa meant going from viewing panic as catastrophic and dangerous to now viewing panic as inconvenient, from virtually intolerable to mildly uncomfortable. The headache overlook intervention was incorporated. This intervention involves three steps: (1) identifying panic symptoms, (2) equating panic with a headache, (3) and beginning to overlook the panic symptoms similarly to the way one would overlook a headache. The goal is for therapists to help clients tolerate anxiety much as they would tolerate a headache. Lisa was able to connect with this intervention and attend to the activities of her daily life while increasingly able to overlook panic feelings and uncomfortable bodily sensations.

Core Pattern	Goal	Intervention(s)
Symptom fears/anxiety sensitivity	Reduce catastrophic misinterpretations	Practice cognitive reappraisals to increase flexibility in appraising situations
Persistent worry about panicking	Reduce worry	Headache overlook intervention
Chronic fear of bodily sensations	Reduce fear	F.E.A.R. – False Evidence that Appears Real; anxiety tolerance

WORRYING VERSUS PROBLEM-SOLVING

Individuals with generalized anxiety disorder struggle with uncontrollable worry. I worked with a man named Bob whose father had Buerger's disease, a recurring progressive inflammation of arteries and veins. Growing up, Bob saw his father get a body part amputated "every time he went to the doctor's." As a result, as a 51-year old man with physical problems, including diabetes, Bob reported that he has been anxious ever since about having to go to the doctor. His worry has worsened since his diabetes has become problematic; his worries trigger panic.

One of the classic strategies for differentiating worrying from problem-solving is the downward arrow technique (Burns, 1980). This involves: (1) identifying the primary worry that is elevating distress, (2) asking the client, "what does this mean about you?" and, (3) continuing the inquiry on the meaning of the worry until an essential belief is reached. In Bob's case, his primary worry was getting sick. *What does that mean about you?* "It would mean that I would have to go to the doctor." *What does that mean about you?* "It would mean that I would get amputated." As the inquiry continued, the amputation eventually meant that he would become "a mean and cruel old man," which is what happened to his father and became his biggest fear and essential belief. This led to problem-solving regarding ways he wasn't going to become a mean and cruel old man regardless of any future physical problems.

PROBLEM-SOLVING HAPPENS IN SMALL STEPS

With worriers, sometimes it is helpful to use a "worry basket." Throughout the day, if Phyllis starts worrying, she stops what she is doing and writes her worry out on a piece of paper. She gradually accumulates these worries and puts them in a basket. At 4:00p.m. each day, she pulls out the worry basket and starts to worry for 30 minutes. For a half-hour, she is asked only to worry. During the day, she gradually teaches herself that the only attention she gives to her worrying is writing down the worry or telling herself that she will have a designated worry half-hour. Writing down the worry teaches Phyllis in a small way to mentally correlate worrying with action.

The second half of the intervention is to take the second half hour (4:30-5:00 p.m.) and problem solve with each identified worry. This involves differentiating what is in the client's control and what is not. And, when doing this task, it is critical that it is the only thing that the client focuses on. Educational research has shown that humans have difficulty simultaneously performing multiple tasks (Ophir, Nass, & Wagner, 2009), despite decades of people's reinforcing the "multitasking myth." This is critical for individuals with GAD because role and task inefficiency is often related to multi-tasking and self-defeating worry.

> *I've missed more than 9,000 shots in my career. I've lost almost 300 games. 26 times, I've been trusted to take the game-winning shot . . . and missed. I've failed over and over and over again in my life. And, that is why I succeed.*
>
> Michael Jordan

PROBLEM-SOLVING IS NOT SOMETHING TO AVOID

Avoidance of problems is a common coping strategy among people with anxiety whereas problem-solving frequently is seen as either monotonous or aversive. Problem-solving is actually the opposite of worrying, and one of the best antidotes to it. When Dawn was worrying about whether she would be accepted into graduate school after all of the applications were sent out, her anxiety continued to elevate, leading to sleep disturbance and decreased appetite. Once she began to problem solve she began to feel a stronger sense of self-control. She ranked her preferred programs and wrote out possible class schedules, specific actions related to moving, and a back-up plan. The more closely the problem-solving addresses the content of the worry, the stronger the sense of control.

Another aspect of problem-solving is probability thinking. When Bill was overwhelmed with driving anxiety because of two accidents in the last three weeks, we collaborated on some arithmetic problems. We estimated that he drove twice a day approximately 350 times a year for 15 years, based on his age and when his regular driving to and from work began. We estimated that he drove 10,500 total times and was accident-free on 10,498 trips. 99.98% of his driving has been accident-free. These numbers helped Bill broaden his perspective and reframe his tunnel vision that had been stuck on only the last three weeks. Probability thinking is a very useful tool in problem-solving worries.

SOCIAL ANXIETY IS EXTREMELY DIFFICULT

Social anxiety is extremely difficult to overcome. DeRubeis, Brotman, & Gibbons (2005) named four psychotherapy treatments matching disorders based on the empirical literature: exposure and response preventions for

Core Pattern	Goal	Interventions
Uncontrollable worry	Challenge worries	Worry basket and problem-solving time; probability thinking
Future orientation	Present-focused objective awareness	Mindfulness exercise Have pt set aside time
Negative cognitive biases	Cognitive restructuring	Downward arrow
Somatic arousal	Reduce arousal and increase tolerance	Diaphragmatic breathing
Role and task inefficiency	Improve efficiency	One task at a time
Social aversiveness	Skills and anxiety	Process relationships

obsessive compulsive disorder, cognitive therapy for panic disorder, exposure therapy for post-traumatic stress disorder (PTSD), and cognitive-behavioral group therapy for social phobia. The latter may be the most difficult, because people with true social anxiety can't stand being in groups. If this describes your clients, they are probably not in the library, coffee shop, or a public restaurant. And, finding somebody to pick up their groceries is a common problem.

TRY THE "NOTICE TALK" ASSIGNMENT

One of my favorite homework assignments for people with social anxiety is what I call the "notice talk" assignment. Patients are asked to go somewhere and stare at something. Then, they ask somebody about something they are staring at (i.e. product on a shelf at a store). If they provide an answer, they say "thank you." Then, they walk away. Patients find this comforting, because there is an "easing-into" effect. They don't engage in eye contact and discomfort is minimal, because all of their attention is on something they are staring at. This notice talk gradually increases.

Another simple strategy is the brown-green technique. Sometimes I ask patients to "notice" everything in my office that is brown. "Try to identify at least 10 things. " After a while, I ask them to close their eyes and try to recall, as much as they can, anything that is green. Some patients can do it but it takes some effort. This simple little intervention is not a life-changing event. It simply makes a point that we are attuned with the brown of life, rather than the green – the life-giving, "go" parts, and the growth of life.

Core Pattern	Goal	Interventions
Self-focused attention	Begin to get outside of self toward talking to others	Brown-green technique, "notice" talk assignment
Negative self-evaluation	Gratitude and improved perception	Count your blessings and connect to personal effort
Anxious apprehension	Improve relaxation skills	Breathing techniques
Avoidance and escape	Increase social activity	Gradual exposure
Skills deficits	Skill building	4-level intervention

INCORPORATING EXPOSURES TO SOCIAL MISHAPS

A key task for therapists to assign clients with social anxiety is gradual mishap exposures. These are situations that are socially anxiety-producing, such as an embarrassing moment or a slip in speech. The goal is to expose the patient to feared consequences by targeting their exaggerated social misperceptions. Sometimes writing a script of how the client will perform a mishap helps reduce avoidance. Essentially, therapists are helping clients confront their fears of negative evaluations from others by teaching them how to make mistakes intentionally. Preparation and post-mishap processing are important for exposure. A mishap script is a set of instructions on how clients can perform three social errors and learn that mishaps are not catastrophic, are tolerable, and are widespread. Here are some examples:

- Stand in front of a restaurant and ask for directions to that restaurant.
- Buy $10.00 worth of groceries with change and drop it all while handing the money to the cashier.
- Trip in front of a group of people.
- Buy a can opener and then immediately return it saying, "I forgot, I already have one."

FOUR-LEVEL INTERVENTION

One of my favorite interventions for social phobia is a modified version of John Buri's (2006) four levels of communication. I began applying these levels in an educational and practical intervention format. Since I began applying this intervention in 2006 at Michigan State University, my patients report increased confidence, improved social skills, and decreased social anxiety. It involves learning the different levels of communication and applying these levels in day to day communications.

Level I communication consists of small talk: "How are you doing?" "What's up?" you know–weather talk. Level II communication consists of people, places, and things talk. This communication centers on people that we know or places that we've gone or plan to go or things that we've learned or done. Level III communication is related to what people reveal about their attitudes, values, and beliefs. This has to do with disclosing personal information about who we are, what's important to us, and what we really care about. When we touch upon this level, we reveal what we believe and what we value. Level IV communication is even more personal and deep. In this level, we begin to share with someone the impact circumstances and events are having on us personally. This involves more than using emoticons on text messages. This entails more than using hashtags with emotion words on tweets. Pokes and message boards are not level IV. True level IV is in-person and very emotionally personal.

Sometimes Containment Is The Goal

When I worked at Hazelden in St. Paul, Minnesota, I worked with addicts in recovery. Many had dual diagnoses, which included mood disorders and anxiety disorders. They needed help in learning containment skills. For them, going to level IV was automatic but learning to speak in level I and II was actually more difficult. One woman named Tamika would attend a family reunion and, when she saw Aunt Ruth, she responded to the "How are you?" question with: "In the last year, I quit my cocaine habit of eight years after I lost my job, and my relationship, and my house went into foreclosure. I found my dog dead in my kitchen due to neglect and my car is totaled." For Tamika, learning to contain her experiences was a necessity. Emotionally vomiting on poor Aunt Ruth was too much. Rapport building necessitates weather talk and chit-chat before emotional disclosure.

Working on a Skills Deficit

People with social anxiety tend to be the opposite of Tamika. They don't have a problem communicating with too much disclosure. They need encouragement to communicate at the basic level and develop from there. And, developing skills takes time and practice. Conceptualizing the communication levels makes it easier. Besides practicing categorizing communication messages within the four levels of communication, the essential goal is for individuals with social anxiety to practice chit-chat and weather talk and begin to develop their social skills. The treatment of social anxiety involves gradual exposure and skill building. Therapists can further help these clients by explaining that time, practice, and patience are needed with notice talk assignments and four-level communication training or other interventions that increase exposure and social skills.

OBSESSIVE-COMPULSIVE DISORDER: GAINING PERSONAL POWER

The goal of OCD treatment is to limit the power of unwanted, repeated, intrusive thoughts, images, and urges. Freedom from fear is largely related to becoming free of fears from within. And, freedom from fears related to obsessions and compulsions results in gaining personal power.

When people are obsessive compulsive about being clean, their power is in being dirty. When people are obsessive compulsive about being perfect, their power is in being imperfect. When people are obsessive compulsive about being certain, their power is in being uncertain. Fully accepting that most parts of life are dirty, imperfect, and uncertain can be life-giving and help clients with OCD increase their personal power. The essential goal of OCD treatment is exposure (to being dirty, imperfect, and uncertain) and not performing the related ritual such as hand-washing (also known as ritual prevention).

Core Pattern	Goal	Interventions
Unwanted, repeated, intrusive thoughts	Limit their power	Tolerance thought
Images		Safe place installation and image replacement
Urges		Tolerance of urge and decision to engage in present-centered activity (increase flow)
Compulsive behavior	Ritual prevention	Exposure and ritual prevention; distraction

CORE PATTERN INTERVENTIONS FOR OBSESSIVE COMPULSIVE DISORDER

A core intervention for intrusive thoughts is increasing tolerance thoughts. This involves reminders that when these thoughts come, they can be tolerated. The essential feature that reinforces OCD is the inability to tolerate uncertainty or randomness. So, naturally, the antidote is the opposite—coming to a place where uncertainty becomes more tolerable. OCD is associated with structural and functional brain abnormalities, particularly in the orbital frontal cortex and basal ganglia (Szeszko et al., 1999; Whiteside, Port, & Abramowitz, 2004). The neuroplasticity of the brain allows these abnormalities to change and decrease as tolerance increases.

> *Decision is a sharp knife that cuts clean and straight; indecision, a dull one that hacks and tears and leaves ragged edges behind it.*
>
> Gordon Graham

Unwanted images need image replacement. These come from the visuals of your life: (1) your favorite place on a beach, (2) a painting of a beautiful scene into which you projected yourself as a child, (3) a mysterious image seared in your memory from the visit you made to Beijing, China. Identify an image from memory. Consider the image and notice the sounds, sights, smells, beauty, and recognize the experience of peace, calm, and tranquility replacing any angst while in this safe place.

Urge replacement involves deciding to engage in activity that produces flow: swimming, aerobic/cardio, horseback riding, climbing, writing poetry near a waterfall, snow-shoeing, reading by a fire, coaching kids, playing poker, practicing handstands and cartwheels (my seven-year old daughter is teaching me these), musky fishing in the north or marlin fishing in the Gulf, or reading. I recently had a client who goes outside and lifts tractor tires to increase her heart rate. The list is endless and the only criterion is that the activity allows you to be so immersed that you aren't thinking; instead, you are engaged.

The primary core intervention in OCD is ritual prevention. To not wash, check, or arrange. This includes not performing behaviors in response to perceived defects in physical appearance such as mirror checking, excessive grooming, or reassurance seeking. This also entails not hoarding, skin-picking (excoriation), or pulling hair (trichotillomania). And distraction helps. In addition to flow activities, intentional plans to distract when obsessions enter the stream of consciousness provide temporary relief. This is usually helpful as a supplemental method for a brief and structured period of time – television, writing a letter, reading Facebook posts; the goal is to prevent rituals. Caution should be taken that distraction activities don't lead to avoidance.

The essential treatment of OCD is exposure and response prevention (Huppert & Roth, 2003). Multiple research studies indicate that between 63% and 83% of participants obtain some benefit following exposure and response prevention, and many gains were maintained over time (Abramowitz, 1997; Foa & Kozak, 1996). OCD treatment is the exact opposite of ADHD treatment. It is interesting to note that the goal of OCD treatment is to not perform rituals whereas the goal of ADHD treatment is to develop beneficial rituals.

Becoming Unafraid Of Memories

A prominent cluster of symptoms for individuals with PTSD includes flashbacks and nightmares. One of the goals of PTSD treatment is to become unafraid of such memories. The thought: "It's happening again" is a common interior source of anxiety. Acceptance, tolerance, and a reality check are helpful in concluding that: *It's not happening again!*

> I learned that courage was not the absence of fear, but the triumph over it. The brave man is not he who does not feel afraid, but he who conquers that fear.
>
> Nelson Mandela

Upon awakening or awareness, a reality check involves recognizing the time, date, and location. Just because it's raining doesn't mean one is in Vietnam. While there is traffic, the car accident was six years ago. Running across this marathon finish line is not the finish at the 2013 Boston Marathon.

Learning To Have Less Guilt

It is common to have all kinds of thoughts of, "I could have done this" or "I should have done that." I talked with a Vietnam Veteran who walked away from his partner at post to smoke a cigarette; within a minute, his partner was shot in the head by a sniper. For decades, "I never should have left my post" resounded in his head.

> Courage is resistance to fear, mastery of fear, not absence of fear.
>
> Mark Twain

In 2004, I spoke with a man who lost his fiancée in a terrible car accident that he survived. He was paralyzed with guilt about how he should have made different decisions as the truck swerved in front of him. "I should have stayed in my lane."

Such guilt sinks deep within a person. The sexual assault survivor blames herself. The wounded warrior is angry at his "missteps." The mother whose son was kidnapped is beset with guilt at having turned her back to talk to a friend at the park.

SELF-DIRECTED EXPOSURE ELEVATES THEN REDUCES

> *Life shrinks or expands in proportion to one's courage.*
>
> Anais Nin

Exposure elevates then reduces anxiety. It is the elevation that often causes avoidance and angst about exposure. On a scale from 0 (complete relaxation) and 10 (maximum anxiety), avoidant veterans experience an 8, 9, or 10 when they drive into a parking lot at the VA. If they drive away without getting out of the car, their anxiety level drops to a 0.

I worked with a college student (let's call her Jane) who shared a story about her mother dying in their house when it burned down. The night it happened, the young woman got in a fight with her mother about going out with her boyfriend. Against her mother's wishes, Jane went out. Upon her return, she found her mother's house was burning down with her mother inside and unable to escape. The horrifying experience, an unimaginable nightmare, occurred in front of her and stayed with her. Her sleep disturbances, depression, intrusive reminders and flashbacks and guilt were intense.

> *God, give us grace to accept with serenity the things that cannot be changed, courage to change the things which should be changed and the wisdom to distinguish the one from the other.*
>
> Reinhold Niebuhr

When Jane made it into my office, her anxiety was a 10. Due to failing relationships and poor grades, she realized that she needed to talk to somebody or she would never be able to move on. The hardest part of therapy was that talking about her trauma elevated her anxiety intensely, but as time went by the anxiety went down. Jane was asked to write out the details of her story from the beginning of her argument with her mother until the end of the night. She was then asked to read the story out loud every day which included audio recording and listening to her reading her story. She did this daily between sessions. Her anxiety rating for each of the next 6 days between sessions was a 10, 10, 9, 7, 4, and 2. When she came in the next week and read the story to me, that is when her emotional intensity elevated with tears, discomfort, and immense sadness. She was surprised how her 2 became a 10. Following the trauma processing, Jane was asked to write out the story again. This time, she was asked to include forgotten details, add more emotion words, and elaborate on sensory details such as images, sounds, sensations, and recalled thoughts. After she wrote out a more extensive story, she then read it again daily over the next week. Jane's anxiety elevated but then came down as expected.

STORY EXPOSURE AND EXPIRING GUILT

There are two goals with someone like Jane: re-exposure to her traumatic memories through telling her story and helping her reduce her guilt. First, story exposure involved asking Jane to write out her story and then read it every day between sessions. Below are the Dos and Don'ts of story exposure.

Do	Don't
Visualize imagery of a safe place before you write and read the story	Approach it like caffeine; don't write or read several hours before bed
Self-soothe with positive self-talk (I can do this)	Don't rush through the story, ignoring the anxiety; feel it
Tell yourself as your anxiety goes up that you can tolerate the distress	Don't avoid the stress
Scale the anxiety by noting a 0 (completely calm) to 10 (maximum anxiety)	Don't just write the facts. As you write your story, include as many descriptive details and emotion words as you can.

As Jane read the story, she would add descriptors and emotions, "Oh, this is what I was feeling," particularly when writing the second account of the story. She read it daily and the anxiety associated with the trauma began to decrease. While the horror of her story remains, with exposure to her memories, her anxiety dissipated. This is the process of healing.

The other goal is to help survivors like Jane with her guilt–the "I should have done this and I should have done that" type of guilt. When these clients are no longer experiencing emotion but are instead able to take an eagle's perspective and look at things in a more objective way is when we practice reappraisals. This involves writing the specific thought: "My mother wouldn't have died if I had stayed at home." After the belief is rated: how much do you believe this thought on a scale of 0-100 (0 completely false, 100 completely true), then we start to challenge the thought. This entails seeking evidence for or against this belief. By the end of this process, Jane concluded that "there were just going to be some things that I will never know," like, maybe whether another set of eyes and ears and another nose would more effectively remedied the problem of the old fire alarm batteries. The guilt beliefs are usually shoulds (i.e., I should have. . .). These shoulds are addressed with the core trauma intervention below using the four steps of cognitive restructuring.

Core Pattern	Goal	Interventions
Fears of memories	Increase present-centered activity, separate past from present; reduce fear of memories	It's not happening again! Acceptance, tolerance and reality check
Trauma memory	Elevate then reduce anxiety associated with memory	Story exposure
Guilt over acts of commission or omission Survivor guilt	Reduce Guilt	Cognitive Restructuring a. Describe the event b. Write thoughts; rate beliefs 0-100%; how much do you believe this thought? c. Challenge thoughts: Evidence for? Evidence against? d. How else can I interpret the event? Rate belief in alternative thought 0-100%

ANXIETY SPIRALS

Anxiety occurs in a spiral of interactions among thoughts, images, physical sensations, emotions, and behaviors. I recently saw Jermaine, a former football and track star from a big time Division 1 university in Florida. He ran the 100-meter dash in 10.4 seconds and had significant playing time in his first two years in college football in the 1980's. He lost his scholarship due to drugs and ended up in and out of prison, incarcerated 10 times over 25 years. Unlike many convicts, he didn't have a personality disorder. Like many convicts, he had to work hard on his substance use disorder. Upon his final release, he began talking to kids at his old high school about not using drugs and described the trajectory of his life that resulted from his choices. He stated that he was channeling his energy toward doing positive things in his life. When I asked him about what he referred to as his "calling" and his sobriety, he would light up. His entire affect came to life. His problem is that this type of motivational speaking is primarily volunteer and not paid. When I ask him about employment, he shuts down which starts his anxiety spiral. When he starts to think about a marketable skill and his resume, his spiral of worries begin to spin in his mind. He has limited work skills and suffers from GAD. He has worry and anxiety spirals about the future, job interviews, and money.

One of the gold nuggets that can be taken from this story is the importance of meanings in our reactions. The meaning a person attaches to an experience accounts for the feelings of anxiety. It is helpful to recognize the link between the worries and the emotional responses. For Jermaine, the link that connected his worry spirals was the fear that his work future was limited. Insight develops for clients when the therapy emphasizes transitions from beliefs about circumstances to beliefs about themselves. Jermaine was asked what he believed about himself due to his work limitations. The meaning he attached to his limitations was "I always fail at everything I try." This was the substance of therapy and Jermaine's spiral stopper going forward. Collaboratively, we began to examine the evidence and consider alternative explanations and empowering meanings.

Every Reaction Results from Two Experiences

The anxiety spiral is a repeated set of these internal experiences at one time over multiple increments of time, creating an onion effect. It is not uncommon for a person living a life of reflection to see that uncovering understanding is a lot like pulling back parts of an onion. Insight takes time because people are naturally absorbed in their circumstances. Understanding beliefs

> An unexamined life is not worth living.
>
> Socrates

about one's self and meanings attached to experiences is hard work. This exploration of the interior life is more like a journey than a destination. If the greatest predictor of future behavior is past behavior, then understanding past behavior is needed if the goal is change.

One helpful truth in the journey of exploring the interior life is that every reaction is either: (1) a classically conditioned response or, (2) an interpretation of an experience. Every reaction is either from a trigger we have learned to respond to or our own "thinking about thinking." Every experience of anxiety is a result of a triggered stimulus or a thread of thoughts.

MANY ANXIETY REACTIONS ARE CLASSICALLY CONDITIONED

When Lisa was raped, the last thing she saw when her lamp was kicked over was sunglasses. On her way to her job at JC Penney a few weeks later, she passed a person wearing sunglasses and she fell to her knees in a panic attack. Since the perpetrator came in through her bedroom window a few blocks from the university campus, opening her window for fresh air was anxiety-producing. Lisa's triggers and scaled anxiety (0-completely relaxed to 10-maximum anxiety) is below.

Trigger	Scaling
Sunglasses	10
Closing her Window	9
Working at JC Penney	7
Selling sunglasses off the racks at work	10

For years, triggers such as gasoline smell or fireworks have elicited anxiety (associated with explosions) for veterans returning from tours. Driving triggers panic for serious car accident survivors. A boat oar is a trigger for a man whose father used it to beat him with it at their summer cabin. A waiting room triggers concerns about humiliation for a person with social phobia. Soap can trigger anxiety about being dirty and subsequent obsessions for a person with obsessive-compulsive disorder. Road kill elicited emotional distress for a veteran who found bombs in dead animals. Driving over pot-holes can be excruciating for veterans who are used to looking for IED's on the sides of the road. A baby's cry may trigger grief for a mother who just had a miscarriage. Somebody yelling may remind a person of his

> Tomorrow hopes we have learned something from yesterday.
>
> John Wayne

or her bipolar parent. For many months after the tragedy, the Columbine principal worked to change the tone and sound of the fire alarm that was going off for hours during the massacre so that it wouldn't elicit terrorizing fear for the kids the next time it went off for a fire drill.

Each person has a list of conditioned stimuli that elicit responses. Songs, perfume, ocean waves, a chocolate covered cherry, the smell of a baby's skin, or a cheering crowd–which now may feel different for 2013 Boston Marathon runners.

The two brain structures crucial for memory formation are the hippocampus, which encodes information in short-term memory, and the amygdala, which is involved with emotional activation. For many of us, an ocean wave keeps the amygdala mildly active or mainly neutral, but if you've lost a child in a drowning, the amygdala becomes extremely activated resulting in an unforgettably painful memory elicited by an ocean wave.

> *If you go against your reinforcement history, you are in for a fight.*
>
> Dr. John Buri

For those triggers that evoke negative emotion, the remedy is exposure. Exposure elevates anxiety (up the scale toward 10) and then brings it down (down the scale toward 0). For individuals facing those triggers that bring on fear, they are in for a fight if they persist in confronting their fears. The key to exposure is readiness. A good therapist will say, "When you are ready, exposure is critical, but not until you are ready."

Most Anxiety Reactions Result from Thinking

Lisa thought a lot about her decision to live near campus. Not in her wildest thought did she foresee an assault. But, three months prior, she had wrestled with the difficult decision of accepting a job closer to home or staying near the university, taking out more loans, and pursuing a master's degree. Against her parents' recommendations, she decided for the latter with the hopes of getting her MBA to better position herself in a challenging economy.

> *If we wish to conquer undesirable emotional tendencies in ourselves, we must ... cold-bloodedly go through the outward motions of those contrary dispositions we prefer to cultivate.*
>
> William James

Since the assault, Lisa has been overwhelmed by guilt and shame. Her regret is intertwined with her obsessions over her job. "Did I make the right decision to come back here?" As Lisa continues to tell herself that she made the wrong decision, her despair deepens. Therapists with expertise in sexual assault and sexual assault nurse examiners (SANEs) train crisis intervention volunteers to communicate: "It's not your fault" to assault survivors. Lisa had heard this but still ruminated about the "things I could have done." Beliefs that elevated Lisa's anxiety include "I am worthless," "I am defective," and "I am unlovable."

Most anxiety comes from our thoughts. For a person with social anxiety, "I will be humiliated in front of others" is one of many thoughts. For a person with post-traumatic stress disorder, "It is happening again," is at the heart of many thoughts. For a person with obsessive-compulsive disorder, "This must be in order," is one of many thoughts. For a person with generalized anxiety disorder, "It will turn out horribly," is an example of one of the more common thoughts. For a person with panic disorder, "I can't stand these feelings," is one of many thoughts.

A common homework assignment is to take some time to differentiate the anxiety-producing triggers and the anxiety-producing thoughts. Triggers can be internal (bodily sensations or flashbacks) and external (sunglasses).

Stimulus / Trigger	Thoughts
Driving in traffic	I will get in another car accident.
Test being handed out	I will not pass the test.
Speaking in class	I will forget what I want to say.
Exercise	I am in terrible shape.
Bodily sensations like shortness of breath	I am going to panic and I will not be able to cope.

ABNORMAL VERSUS NORMAL ANXIETY

Everybody gets anxious. When someone returns to a dentist after no appointments for 10 years, their anxiety is understandable. People often make themselves nervous prior to family reunions. Professional athletes who have played the game their entire lives report routine anxiety. Dave Novicki, anxiety specialist at Michigan State University Counseling Center, often tells patients: "You want anxiety when you are walking in the middle of the street, because you will get out of the way when a truck is coming." Anxiety around having a snake loose in your car is normal (and fear is automatic). The question is – what type of anxiety is normal and what anxiety is abnormal? An important related question is identifying the goal of treatment. I tell therapy clients that the goal isn't to eliminate anxiety. The goal is to make the anxiety manageable.

Abnormal anxiety is different from normal anxiety in that it involves cognitive distortions. These are usually erroneous danger appraisals (Beck et al., 1985). I notice that clients with panic disorder, who are frequently afraid of having panic attacks tend

> *Self-searching is the means by which we bring new vision, action, and grace to bear upon the dark and negative side of our nature. With it comes the development of a kind of humility... We find that bit by bit we can discard the old life – the one that did not work – for a new life that can and does work.*
>
> As Bill Sees It

to distort their cognitions in a similar pattern. It may look different and follow a different psychological sequence with different symptoms, but it tends to start with tunnel vision. Shortness of breath may trigger tunnel vision, which involves zooming in on the symptom like a laser beam. Then magnification of the symptom leads to other symptoms. As chest discomfort, accelerated heart rate, a feeling of choking, and dizziness start (DSM-5 criteria for a panic attack involves four of 13 symptoms) then catastrophizing begins. This involves the thought that a panic attack will be a catastrophe. This results in a discrete period of intense fear or discomfort.

Abnormal anxiety is also associated with impaired functioning. Life essentially comes down to work and relationships, and these are the areas that abnormal anxiety affects. Rape survivors are reported to experience a physical paralysis (Barlow, 2002). Triggers, or reminders, can be so strong in the level of anxiety that is elicited, that work and relationships are like a movie that has been permanently paused by a broken remote. For some, their bodily memories are frozen in time, usually stuck at the time when the anxiety originated.

FALSE ALARMS AND STIMULUS HYPERSENSITIVITY

Abnormal anxiety is also associated with false alarms (Barlow, 2002). When I speak at seminars, it is common for conference room staff to fill the water pitchers. Most of us don't have a second thought about a water pitcher unless you had a recent experience of your drunk cousin showing up at your sister's wedding and dumping a pitcher of water on you as you tried to break up a wedding quarrel. But, false alarms occur outside of external triggers. A small sense of fear related to losing control or a whispering thought of uncertainty can arouse the alarms. Individuals with abnormal anxiety develop stimulus hypersensitivity, a fear that is elicited by situations of relatively mild threat intensity that would usually be perceived as harmless to a non-fearful person (Beck & Greenberg, 1988). So, a catastrophic misinterpretation of a pitcher of water or an increased heart rate (for example following exercise) can be reflective of stimulus hypersensitivity.

THE TWO MOST COMMON ANXIOUS THREADS

The two most common forms of anxious thinking or cognitive distortions are emotional reasoning and catastrophizing. Emotional reasoning is what Jason is doing when he tells himself that he is a failure because he avoided the interview again. Thinking rationally is difficult when we are in an anxiety spiral, because of the amygdala's hijacking of the neocortex. In these situations, the amygdala, the emotional center of the brain, overwhelms the neocortex and impairs the person's ability to think logically (Ledoux, 1996). Psychiatrist Daniel Siegel calls this "flipping our lids," because the frontal cortex (our brain's "lid") has lost its ability to control limbic system physiology and maintain amygdala regulation (Siegel & Hartzell, 2003).

The amygdala is the key structure for processing fear, anxiety, and other states of emotional arousal. Using functional magnetic resonance imaging (fMRI), we can see significantly increased brain activity in the area of the amygdala during a panic attack. During this experience, people often experience a "flooding" of emotion. The idea of flooding was originally suggested by psychologist Paul Ekman who was a pioneer in the study of emotion and human facial expressions (1984).

Catastrophizing in the thought life works similarly to flooding in the emotional life. When a dashboard light comes on in Jerry's car, the flooding of emotion leads him to perceive an inconvenience as a disaster. With the sympathetic nervous system acting as the body's accelerator, overwhelming emotion leads a person like Jerry to fail to reinterpret life contexts in calm and realistic ways (it would take activation of the parasympathetic system to act as the body's brakes in order for a calm, realistic interpretation).

Consider a clip from the 1984 film, *Footloose*, Ren's friends tie his shoelaces around the accelerator during a tractor chicken game to prevent him from jumping off the moving tractor. During emotional flooding, sympathetic activity works in a similar way. Sympathetic activity involves experiencing constant acceleration leading an anxious individual to perceive inconveniences as disasters, scraped knees as broken bones, muscle aches as heart attacks, and difficult but potentially tolerable experiences as catastrophes.

Below is a set of anxiety decatastrophizers, which allow the prefrontal lobes to exert cognitive control over the intense emotionality emanating from the amygdala. In a review of 11 neuroimaging studies, cognitive behavioral therapy was shown to alter functioning in the medial prefrontal cortices, the anterior cingulate, the posterior cingulate and other brain regions associated with problem-solving, self-referential processing, and emotional regulation (Frewen, Dozois, & Lanius, 2008). Cognitive therapy, at its core, involves decatastrophizing perceptions of experiences that appear to be a catastrophe when they usually are nothing more than an inconvenience. A good therapy principle consists of identifying each of these perceptions and differentiating inconveniences from true catastrophes.

Having a panic attack, being perceived as awkward in a social situation, failing a driver's licensing exam, and the washing machine breaking are not catastrophes. These are largely emotional, social, or practical inconveniences. In working with patients to help them differentiate a catastrophe from a mere inconvenience, it is important for the therapist to show compassion, patience, and unconditional positive regard, because what may seem small perturbations from the therapist's perspective still loom large for the patient.

> *The secret to happiness is freedom ... And the secret to freedom is courage.*
>
> Thucydides

Beck et al. (1985, 2001) explain the use of decatastrophizing as modifying exaggerated threat appraisals. It essentially involves identifying the "worst case scenario" and talking about its likelihood, consequences, and the patient's self-perceived ability to cope. What if you did vomit in front of the class? Could you handle it? What if you did fall flat and she didn't want to go on a second date with you? Could you tolerate it?

> *As life goes on, we discover that certain thoughts sustain us in defeat, or give us victory, and it is these thoughts, tested by passion, that we call convictions.*
>
> W. B. Yeats

A DECATASTROPHIZING TECHNIQUE

1. Describe the feared worst-case scenario in as much detail as possible.

2. Ask questions such as: "What is the worst that can happen?" "What is so bad about that?" "What is the most unpleasant part of this worst-case scenario?"

3. Once the scenario is described in detail, assess the likelihood or probability of this scenario actually happening. This involves gathering evidence to further evaluate the likelihood of this scenario.

4. The therapist and the client develop an alternative/more realistic scenario after reviewing the evidence.

5. Seek strengths and gather evidence to increase the client's perceived ability to cope with the more realistic outcome.

CHAPTER 2

Laser Beam Interventions

ANXIETY FOG

Many anxiety problems invade the consciousness like a fog. And, anxiety can have a multiplicative and compounding effect to the problems of life. There are a number of issues that are common among all anxiety problems. While Chapter 1 emphasized differences among anxiety disorders, this chapter emphasizes similarities among anxiety problems. Ten "laser beam" interventions have been identified to address each of the primary problems identified in anxiety:

> *Focus like a laser beam.*
>
> President Bill Clinton

- catastrophizing
- elevating the probability and severity of threats
- unhealthy anxiety anticipation
- self-defeating social beliefs
- fear of anxiety symptoms
- limited internal and external resources
- intolerance of uncertainty
- comfort zone dependence
- chronic worry
- external locus of control

CATASTROPHIC MISINTERPRETATIONS ARE COMMON

Janet has fibromyalgia, diabetes, and chronic obstructive pulmonary disorder (COPD). She is working hard to control her diabetes through her diet but is having difficulty getting exercise due to joint pain. Her breathing difficulties add to her problems. On top of these physical problems, Janet has struggled

25

with panic disorder for four years, and she has an intense fear of having more panic attacks and losing control ("going crazy"). Research indicates that clients with panic disorder are susceptible to catastrophically misinterpreting uncomfortable bodily sensations (Hoehn-Saric, McLeod, Funderburk, & Kowalski, 2004; McNally & Foa, 1987).

Janet began to make progress with her anxiety when she enhanced her cognitive reappraisal capabilities. Cognitive reappraisal decreases the amygdala's emotional responses. She began to see her anxiety symptoms differently by developing multiple interpretations of her own symptoms, and she began to have more realistic explanations of her bodily sensations. She began to be able to differentiate between catastrophes and mere inconveniences. She also started to view her panic sensations the way she sees a headache, uncomfortable, but not HORRIFIC.

Laser Beam	Action
Weaken catastrophic misinterpretations	Practice reappraisals of symptoms

Janet's threat was her physical, bodily sensations. She had a fear of having panic attacks, of dying ("heart attack"), and losing control. She also had a fear of fainting, which is actually quite rare, because it requires a significant drop in blood pressure. Janet established more benign and realistic explanations for her symptoms–that she wasn't going to die or lose control. She began to realize that as she experienced uncomfortable bodily sensations, she could maintain control. She also began to practice a 3-step cue sequence that would remind her to reinterpret her bodily sensations. When she noticed nausea or an accelerated heart rate, she would remember that, "this is a catastrophe" was one possible interpretation of her symptoms. She would initiate the sequence by counting slowly to five and taking deep breaths. The deep breaths would involve saying "in" for three seconds and "out" for three seconds as she breathed in and out. Step 2 would involve touching her ear as a physical cue and a reminder to practice reappraisals. Step 3 involves thinking through three appraisals of her own bodily sensations. Examples of reappraisals would include interpreting the sensations as "an opportunity to apply my learned coping strategies" or '"like an unpleasant headache" or an experience "to accept and tolerate while going on with my day."

CLIENTS NEED MOORINGS

Clients are often on a boat blown around by the waves of life influenced by the currents and the winds from stressful life events. In boating, a mooring is a permanent structure that secures a vessel. In life, clients often are without moorings. Yet they need moorings to help them stabilize when the stressors of life are overwhelming.

> *We are all in the same boat, in a stormy sea, and we owe each other a terrible loyalty.*
>
> G. K. Chesterton

In therapy sessions, structure and agenda setting can help reduce overwhelm. Agenda setting involves identifying a beginning and an ending with the first five minutes following brief chit-chat focused on the 2, 3, or 4 issues to be discussed. Also, five minutes are saved at

> *All of us need to grow continuously in our lives.*
>
> Les Brown

the end of the session to discuss how therapy went, how the therapist did, what was missed, and what was remembered as a valuable component of the session.

In addition to setting an agenda for the session, certain types of mental clarity provide moorings. One of the strong winds causing anxiety hardship is perceptions of elevated threat and danger and the perceived severity of those threats. Scaling is an efficient way to identify the level of threat and a person's perceived ability to cope with the stressful situation. What is the probability of the threat (some "bad" outcome) happening –0 (unlikely) to 10 (likely)? What is the severity of this event – 0 (not severe) to 10 (catastrophic)? The most important scaling question is assessing a client's perception of their ability to cope with a stressor. On a scale of 0 – 10, what is your perception of your ability to cope with this threat? Or, in your perception, what is the strength of your coping at this time (0-10)?

Laser Beam	Action
Scaling X3	Use probability, severity, and coping scaling

MODIFYING THREAT APPRAISALS REDUCES FEAR

The goal of modifying threat appraisals has two parts: (1) interpreting situations more realistically and (2) increasing one's perception of coping. When a college student has speaking anxiety and manages to gut out a speech, he is likely going to interpret his recent speech as "bad" and his ability to "gut it out" as poor. Over time, the college student may reinterpret the event and start to see how the speech did go well at least in some ways. A job interview, a sales pitch, a date, a fishing expedition, or learning to ride a bike can all depend on interpretation.

Re-interpreting is particularly important for evaluating the success of anxiety management. In treatment using cognitive behavioral therapy, when the client is ready, he or she is often encouraged to undertake actions that will require courage. For example, a veteran anxious about driving over pot holes may be encouraged to drive over pot holes when he is ready. If he is unable to complete this action, but instead is forced by his anxiety to pull over, he needs to understand that his categorizing his efforts as a failure is unhelpful. The goal is for him to re-interpret his efforts so that he can begin to perceive his courage and resilience in the face of reminders of death. The veteran may perceive success if he drove over the pot holes and failure if he pulled over. Re-interpreting the dichotomous thinking toward incremental and small successes is helpful. Success and strength finding is then focused on what the client did do (e.g. driving a part of the way or at least giving it consideration). This process strengthens the veteran's perception of coping when courageously facing triggers.

ANTICIPATING ANXIETY INCREASES FEARLESSNESS WITH GENERATED ALTERNATIVES

One of the best ways to increase fearlessness is to anticipate when you will get anxious. People with fear and anxiety tend to anticipate well, which is why they have particular safety-seeking behaviors that reinforce anxiety. Some people will only go grocery shopping with a drawn out map of a grocery store with a written arrow of each aisle they will go to. Others will only go places with their bottle of Xanax. Some will even take their empty bottles of Xanax.

> *The paradox of our time in history is that we have taller buildings, but shorter tempers; wider freeways, but narrower viewpoints; we spend more, but have less; we buy more, but enjoy it less.*
>
> George Carlin

One of the comments that I make to clients all of the time is that "anxiety will go up." This way it is never a surprise when they return to therapy with anxiety shooting up to an 8, 9, or a 10. Anticipating increased arousal leads a person to rely on safety-seeking behaviors (YOUR LINUS BLANKET). It also leads a person to develop a plan about how to cope. Generating alternatives in social situations is one way to deal, without depending on safety-seeking behaviors. Clients are asked to provide three scenarios with one of them based on how they usually act in a similar situation–avoidant, fearful, non-communicative, indifferent and with poor eye contact. Then I ask: "What are two additional scenarios that you can generate for how you might respond more effectively in this upcoming social situation?" Here is an example of an alternative interpretation for an upcoming social situation–"I can feel anxious and still be competent in social situations."

Laser Beam	Action
Anticipatory anxiety reduction intervention	Generate alternatives in anticipating upcoming anxiety- producing social situations

MODIFYING THREAT APPRAISALS IS ESSENTIALLY SHOWING "BEND" IN OUR BELIEF

Our time in life basically comes down to work and relationships. Most anxiety is related to these two areas. It is common for people with anxiety to be rigid in their beliefs, particularly about relationships. Showing clients how to "bend" helps them to see that beliefs can shift. Sometimes in life we experience insights or epiphanies that allow us to see something new about ourselves. When this happens, something new enters, but something already present within ourselves begins to change. In rare moments, this can happen within therapy. I worked with a man named Omot who struggled with feelings of helplessness and powerlessness. Omot was an immigrant from Ethiopia. He held a college degree and had spent many years in the U.S. He used his political science degree in his writing about Ethiopian politics but he felt underemployed as a cook in a restaurant. He had particular difficulty with a co-worker who repeatedly stated, "You don't belong here." Whenever this stressor occurred, it would remind him of old beliefs – that he was helpless and powerless. Over time, he was able to see that these were only beliefs and that they could shift. First, in collaboration, we identified the core beliefs of "I am helpless" and "I am powerless." During evidence gathering, we identified experiences of Omot's personal power: escaping a war torn part of his country, moving to the United States with his spouse, pursuing and graduating from college, and traveling throughout the world. It became clear that Omot was trapped in the "absorbed in circumstances" phenomenon. As he began to take a broader perspective of his life, the helpless belief about his coworker situation minimized in his mind. "Now this problem seems so small." The most important part of therapy was that he began to see that his belief could change, or bend. Omot began to see that his belief in his powerlessness could begin to change toward seeing himself as empowered and powerful.

WHAT DO YOU WANT TO BELIEVE ABOUT YOURSELF?

A person is empowered when he or she becomes aware of self-defeating beliefs: "I am inadequate in an interview;" "I am helpless due to my social anxiety;" I am incompetent when I am around women." When these self-defeating beliefs are scaled from 0 (I believe it is completely false) to 10 (I believe it is completely true), it is common for these self-defeating beliefs to be rated as closer to the true end of the scale.

It is difficult initially for many clients with social anxiety to believe the following: "I am adequate in interviews;" "I am able to cope with my social anxiety;" "I am competent around women." I do not ask clients to believe this or tell them that they should believe this. Rather I ask: "What do you want to believe about yourself in social situations? What would need to happen for you to believe that about yourself?"

Laser Beam	Action
Scaling validity of cognitions in social situations	On a scale of 0 (completely false) to 10 (completely true), how true is this belief about you now?

BECOMING TOLERANT AND UNAFRAID

Individuals with trauma in their backgrounds are often afraid of certain experiences due to hypervigilance which they have developed to protect themselves. This includes perceiving threats from things that most people would view as harmless. Consider a cash register used regularly at restaurants and businesses. Most of us wouldn't think twice about this benign stimulus unless we had worked the cash register at a gas station and were a victim of a robbery. The "benign" cash register is now a negative memory producer.

> I am only one, but I am one. I cannot do everything, but I can do something. And I will not let what I cannot do interfere with what I can do.
>
> Edward Everett Hale

Similarly, an assault survivor may have triggered sensations from sunglasses if they were the last object she saw prior to the rape. Veterans hit the deck during the 4th of July fireworks because they associate these sounds and flashes of light with warfare. The smell of gasoline at the gas pump elicits fears for the survivor of the helicopter crash. The song being played at the mall may remind a woman whose boyfriend was killed.

It Is More than Just Triggers

Anxiety results from more than just triggers. Sunglasses, fireworks, gasoline smells, and songs evoke distressing emotion. The goal of treatment is to confront these triggers rather than avoid them. In the end, the goal for therapists is to help clients not have anything control their lives.

> *The greatest artists like Dylan, Picasso and Newton risked failure. And if we want to be great, we've got to risk it too.*
>
> Steve Jobs

The "perceived threat" involves more than just reminders of past traumatic experiences. The most difficult core symptom is being afraid of memories. Becoming *tolerant* and *unafraid* of traumatic memories is at the heart of the T & U intervention.

The T & U Intervention Requires Three Steps

Becoming tolerant and unafraid requires three steps: strength building, facing triggers, and cognitive restructuring. To restructure, reflection on these two questions builds M&M's (Mental Muscle): In what ways can you tolerate these symptoms? In what ways are you unafraid of these symptoms?

Laser Beam	Action
T & U intervention	In what ways can you tolerate these symptoms? In what ways are you unafraid of these symptoms?

Increasing Resourcefulness in Adversity

A common problem for individuals struggling with anxiety is that they maintain the perception that they have limited resources in the face of adversity. This includes perceiving limitations on both internal and external resources. Perceiving internal limitations involves disbelief that they can handle turmoil, cope with difficulty, or work through relationship conflicts. External resource limitations involve believing others aren't going to be there for them. Even if support is great, what is perceived through the anxiety lens is isolation.

A key intervention in cognitive behavioral therapy is evidence gathering. This involves the therapist helping a client gather evidence for how they are a strong and resourceful person. The following are evidence-seeking questions about internal strength and resources.

- In what ways have you demonstrated inner strength in the face of adversity?
- What milestones are you proudest about or most grateful for and in what ways did you show strength during those experiences?

For a broader perspective, the therapist helps the client objectively view the evidence:

- What is the evidence that you manage adversity halfheartedly?
- What is the evidence that you manage adversity with strength? Evidence gathering about external resources is essential as well.

Laser Beam	Action
Evidence gathering	Seeking evidence for being a strong and resourceful person

REDUCING INTOLERANCE OF UNCERTAINTY

If "it's happening again" is at the heart of trauma, intolerance of uncertainty is at the heart of obsessive-compulsive problems. Common among obsessive-compulsive disorders, trichotillomania (hair-pulling), hoarding, or excoriation (skin picking) is great distress over uncertainty. People who have these types of problems, are frequently uncomfortable without life guarantees. Uncertainty can paralyze them and rob them of any confidence. Only a small amount of doubt can render them unable to act.

EMBRACING UNCERTAINTY

If the bottom line in OCD and related anxiety disorders, is distress and utter intolerance of uncertainty, then the treatment goal is to increase tolerance of uncertainty. How does a therapist accomplish this with a client? Here are some questions for reflection that increase confidence with uncertainty and reduce efforts to control everything:

- In what ways can you give your opinion even when you aren't certain?
- In what ways could you be more open to surprises in your life?
- In what ways can you be less unhappy when you are uncertain?
- In what ways can you tell yourself "I'm ok with uncertainty" before you go to bed?

- How can you be more flexible with being undecided about your future?
- How can you embrace, rather than avoid, uncertain situations?

Laser Beam	Action
Cognitive restructuring – aimed at reducing efforts to control	Need for IU (intolerance of uncertainty) reframing Learning to embrace uncertainty

EMBRACING UNCERTAINTY REQUIRES LETTING GO

When they are feeling unsure, Lisa may pull her hair, Phil may pick his skin, and Jerry may go to default mode and engage in excessive cleaning. The ritual or "default mode" may be unique, but the distress and anxiety prior to the compulsive behavior is similar. The thing that is aggravating is uncertainty about a problem, uncertain but possible bad news, or something unpredictable that is unresolved. Embracing uncertainty is the first of the battle. Learning to let go is the second part.

Uncertainty consists of many things. A common pattern is feeling the need to control thoughts. This is reinforced by thoughts of needing to be in control (with others or circumstances) or the need to be perfect. Letting go of control and letting go of being perfect is easier said than done, but brings relief from an unnecessarily heavy burden. Here are questions that are at the center of letting go:

- What areas in your life are difficult to let go?
- Which area is most difficult to let go?

Letting go brings great relief. People who obsess about staying clean require help in letting go of the anxiety connected with being dirty. People who obsess about order require help in letting go of the fear of things being out of order. Perfectionists find relief when they can get let go of feeling they need to be perfect.

Laser Beam	Action
Letting-go intervention	What areas in your life are difficult to let go? Which is most difficult to let go?

LETTING GO HELPS WITH WORRIES

Worriers struggle with their chronic worry. They are often conflicted. Part of them wants to worry less; the other part may feel a need to worry to be prepared for possible danger. Therapists make headway when they help them examine the advantages of letting go of the worries. It is important to help the client accept the reality that worry doesn't prepare them for anything.

NORMALIZING WORRY

When college students worry, most worries are normal and similar to the mental experience of other college students. Generally, college students worry about their (1) future, (2) landing a job after graduation, and (3) relationships. Of course, #3 is divided into (a) missing Mom, (b) missing friends, (c) making new friends, (d) possible intimacy

> *In your life you only get to do so many things and right now we've chosen to do this, so let's make it great.*
>
> Steve Jobs

and sexuality – just to name a few. It is common for middle-aged adults to worry about (1) retirement, (2) job stability, and (3) children. It is common for older adults to worry about (1) death, (2) physical limitations, and (3) loneliness.

Normalizing attempts to express the understanding that problem situations are merely a result of being human. This involves acceptance of the client and communicating respect and compassion. The most common and simple sayings that indicate that things aren't as pathological as clients may fear include phrases like "unsurprisingly," "that's often the case," and "of course." In facing particular problems, examples of normalizing include, "many parents might say 'welcome to the club'" or "that's often the case for people when they are faced with the challenge of dealing with such as a difficult boss." Normalizing acknowledges vulnerability to life problems while reframing the notion that the client is alone.

WORRY INDUCTION

In addition to normalizing worries, it is helpful to have clients imagine the worst possible scenario. Essentially, this involves visualizing the many ways in which a particular worry would be a catastrophe. I recently gave a stress management seminar to teachers in a K-8 private school. One of the anxiety-producing problems teachers have to deal with is over-involved "helicopter" parents who yield power with their donations. When a helicopter parent hears that her daughter is bored in science, rather than teach her daughter boredom reduction skills, it is common nowadays for parents to complain to the teacher. Upon hearing about a complaint from the "high powered" mother, the teacher starts to worry about her job. In this scenario, an experimental worry induction involves talking through with the teacher the worst-case scenario. So what would be the worst outcome in this scenario?

1. The parent complains to the principal.

Then what?

2. The principal uses this information in my evaluation and evaluates me negatively.

Then what? What would be the catastrophic outcome in this situation?

3. I get fired.

Then what?

4. I can't pay for my apartment because getting another job would be difficult.

Then what?

5. I have to move home to Connecticut and live in my Grandpa's basement.

Then what?

6. I'd be a loser. I'd feel worthless about my life.

Could you handle that scenario?

7. No, it would be awful. But, I could probably tolerate it. I wouldn't die if that is what you are asking.

WHAT IS THE MORE REALISTIC LIKELIHOOD?

After a client believes that they could cope with the worst-case scenario that would be "catastrophic," the more realistic scenario is considered. After reviewing the more realistic scenario, solutions would be explored regarding how a client would proceed in terms of coping with non-preferred outcomes.

THE RP3 INTERVENTION SOLVES WORRIES

The RP3 intervention starts with identifying worries and then ranking them from most anxiety-producing to least anxiety-producing. After the ranking, then each problem is seen as not (1) *permanent,* (2*) pervasive,* or (3) *personal* (Seligman, 1996).

When Larry lost his job, it was critical that he saw his current job status as temporary, *not permanent.* When Jermaine was cut from his 8th grade baseball team, it was helpful to see that this problem was specific to baseball, *not pervasive* to his other interests or his potential. When Lisa came to see her father's controlling behavior as *his problem,* she began to work through her interior dialogue to separate herself from her father and experience healing; Lisa saw her family of origin problem as empowering *not personal.*

> *Courage does not always roar. Sometimes courage is the quiet voice at the end of the day saying, "I will try again tomorrow."*
>
> Mary Ann Radmacher

Laser Beam	Action
Apply the RP3 intervention	Rank worries; problems are not permanent, but temporary; not pervasive, but specific; not personal, empowering

A LOT OF WORRY "SEEMS UNCONTROLLABLE"

Some people worry all of the time about money or about their job. Others worry constantly about getting in or out of a relationship. Worriers typically believe that life seems out of control and unpredictable. This is often a result of one's thoughts and emotions being influenced by an external locus of control.

Locus of control refers to the extent to which individuals believe that they can control events that influence their lives (Rotter, 1954). A person's "locus of control" is either internal (the person believes they can control their life) or external (meaning they believe that their life is controlled by environmental factors which they cannot influence; like rolling the dice).

College students with an external locus of control who worry may think grades depend entirely on their professor. Job applicants perceive that obtaining work depends entirely on luck. Workers believe that success depends on getting the "right breaks" in life. Finding the "right relationship" depends on being on the right place at the right time. Life is like getting a coin to flip favorably or the dice to roll in the right direction.

CHANGING WORRY FROM UNCONTROLLABLE TO USEFUL

Changing worry from uncontrollable to useful worrying involves adopting an internal locus of control. One of the greatest gifts a therapist can instill within their clients is the all-powerful "INTERNAL LOCUS OF CONTROL!" Consider the aforementioned examples:

College students who worry may think grades depend entirely on their professor. INTERNAL LOCUS OF CONTROL → College students who worry about their grades realize that it depends entirely on their effort.

Job applicants perceive that obtaining work depends entirely on luck. INTERNAL LOCUS OF CONTROL → Job applicants perceive that obtaining work depends on their level of effort.

> *That moment we believe that success is determined by an ingrained level of ability as opposed to resilience and hard work, we will be brittle in the face of adversity.*
>
> Joshua Waitzkin

Workers require getting the "right breaks" in life. INTERNAL LOCUS OF CONTROL → Workers can do well with enough effort, preparation, and determination.

Finding the "right relationship" depends on being at the right place at the right time. INTERNAL LOCUS OF CONTROL → Finding the "right relationship" doesn't depend on fate, but on confidence and a definite course of action.

Life is like getting a coin to flip favorably or the dice to roll in your direction. INTERNAL LOCUS OF CONTROL → What happens to me is based on my own actions, my own plans, and my own effort.

Many worries result from an underlying set of beliefs that derive from a person's locus of control. The intervention consists of an (1) educating the client on locus of control, (2) applying locus of control to specific examples, (3) identifying these examples as external or internal locus of control, (4) generating possibilities on increasing one's internal locus of control.

Laser Beam	Action
U X 2 intervention	Uncontrolled to useful worrying via increasing internal locus of control

CHAPTER 3

Healing From Trauma

There are a variety of responses to traumatization. In this chapter, trauma is characterized as small t or big T. Human unresolved responses to trauma (HURTS) such as self-centeredness, insecurity resulting from attachment problems, inconsistency in relationships, cynicism, and disagreeableness are HURTS explored in this chapter. These responses result in a range of relationship patterns.

In PTSD treatment, therapists need to provide clients with matching remedies for each of their PTSD symptoms. Trauma processing and healing, mindfulness, dissociation treatment, guiding therapy into the therapeutic zone, and positive psychology interventions are all part of the comprehensive treatment package.

BOTH TYPES OF TRAUMA AFFECT NEURAL CIRCUITRY

There are two types of trauma: small ts and big Ts. Both can result in anxiety, fear, worry, social withdrawal, work avoidance, and depression. Both types of trauma can get locked in emotionally and then be triggered because of unprocessed emotion. Thoughts, emotional states, and behavior are influenced by the accumulation of personal experience and memory networks from the past due to this unprocessed emotion.

The Hebbian theory, developed by Donald Hebb in 1949, describes how unprocessed emotion links to memory networks. The adage "neurons that fire together, wire together" summarizes his theory and remains a relevant theory in neuroscience today. Memories form when a stimulus activates the linkage from one neuron to a functionally related neuron. The reverberating electrical activity in neuronal circuits results in short-term memory that consolidates into a long-term memory. Biologists call this memory consolidation long-term potentiation.

The more strongly the neurons fire together, such as in trauma memory, the greater the consolidation and long-term reverberation effect. The limbic system is involved in memory consolidation, storage, and retrieval as well as giving emotional meaning to sensory input. Trauma impact and subsequent symptoms appear due to memory processes that are linked to unprocessed emotions.

Reminders, triggers, emotions, thoughts and feelings of inadequacy can all elicit locked-in emotion that settled in the emotional life of the limbic system and hippocampus due to trauma. Often, these experiences stay with us for a long time because of the strength of the synapses – the way the trauma memory and emotion get stuck together in storage. Sometimes these memories are even locked-in as bodily memories which explains why activities like yoga or massage can bring emotional release. Freedom from fear also includes freedom from memories that entangle and tie people up emotionally.

SMALL TRAUMAS IMPAIR US EMOTIONALLY

Small ts include difficult encounters with others that impact or impair us emotionally. Unfortunately, unless a small t exam of emotional history is completed, people continue to react emotionally to relationship dynamics without realizing or understanding what is setting them off. "My father would make comments almost every day: 'You're fat,' 'How can you be so stupid,' and 'you can never do it right.'"

I recently worked with a 52-year old plumber who was solid at his job. But, he had difficulty talking with people socially. He reported heart palpitations and chest pressure in social situations, particularly at family reunions and get-togethers. He revealed that his father told him, "You will never amount to anything." In 2013, I asked a group of seminar attendees in New Hampshire if they had ever had a client who reported that his or her father had said, "you will never amount to anything;" 48% of therapists raised their hands. When I was in Vermont, 64% of therapists raised their hands to the same question. Clearly, this is a common small trauma that many people have experienced.

A small t examination of emotional history helps to buffer and protect people from reacting out of their Human Unresolved Responses to Trauma (HURTS). These HURTS are emotional and behavioral tendencies that prevent freedom in relating and personal identity. HURTS result from a history of small ts that tend to trap people emotionally. There are a number of HURTS, but let's take a look at some of the frequent HURTS that affect relationships with other people: self-centeredness, insecurity, inconsistency, cynicism, and disagreeableness. For the purpose of synthesizing research data as a book that is primarily evidence-based, it is important to note that this list is not all-inclusive.

Self-Centered People Aren't Necessarily Narcissistic

People who come across as self-centered may actually be inhibited by social anxiety. Often, people who seem obsessed with themselves are actually so worried about how they come across that it impairs them socially. Such people often hear the comment after they warm up (a few years later), "You used to be so arrogant." Their seeming self-absorption, which actually arose from social anxiety, had an unintended effect on their relationships of which they may not have been aware.

On the other hand, sometimes apparent self-centeredness or narcissism isn't a problem of social anxiety. I once worked with a college student named Mark who came in with the presenting problem: "My friends tell me I'm self-centered." He was a delightful young man to talk to – idealistic, optimistic, and witty. Yet some of his behaviors – putting himself first and only caring about his own needs and wants have had some consequences. During our talks, a review of Mark's small ts revealed that his father's comment, "You're not worth my attention" stung him more than any other negative interaction he could remember. He overcompensated with extreme self-care leading to self-centered behavior. In other words, since his father was determined to be unaware of his son, Mark became acutely self-aware and subsequently focused on himself.

Therapists can take time to discuss self-centeredness in therapy. A goal may involve understanding the origin of this behavior. The primary goal is to understand the current impact on relationships in the here and now and to bring about change.

Insecurity Impairs Relationships

Some people have trouble laughing at themselves. Self-deprecating humor is often a nice strategy for helping people feel comfortable and reducing social barriers. Most people like being around people with self-deprecating humor; it helps people ease into conversations. But people with great insecurity are impaired in their ability to authentically connect with others whether it's through humor or other forms of transparency.

Insecurity can start early in life. Let's take a detour and review some of the classic attachment research and theory: Research suggests that parenting styles can influence insecurity. Essentially, a deficit of love is related to a deficit of security. Basically, children who are not sufficiently nurtured become insecure.

> *I'm interested in the fact that the less secure a man is, the more likely he is to have extreme prejudice.*
>
> Clint Eastwood

More specifically, children who are rejected or experience insensitivity from their parents are apt to be insecure, avoidant children who do not seek their attachment figure when distressed (Ainsworth, 1978). Children who experience inconsistency from their parents become insecure, ambivalent, and resistant. They become clingy yet rejecting. They are difficult to soothe, and have difficulty exploring (Ainsworth, 1970). In contrast, securely attached children are the result of consistent responsiveness, warmth, and receptive parenting. As adults, therapists see clients with avoidant attachment styles who tend to be critical and apathetic, and clients with anxious attachment styles who are relationally anxious. Such individuals are frequently troubled by concerns ranging from, "this person doesn't like me" to worries that their feelings won't be reciprocated.

One of the classic attachment models is John Bowlby's internal working model, which involves an internal model of cognitive processes. Based on early attachments, people interpret contact with others based on memories and relational connections from previous emotional and relational exchanges (Bretherton, & Munholland, 1999). Basically, if you have a deficit of love, you will perceive others through that lens. The primary caregiver acts as a prototype for future relationships (Bowlby, 1969), and the internal working model can influence secure versus insecure relationships.

I recently worked with a 28-year old woman named Tamika who never pursued college even though this was something she always wanted to do. She had three children in her early 20s and now feels limited in her possibilities. She came across as socially anxious, tentative, hypersensitive to being evaluated negatively, and fragile. Yet, she had good insight, and she described herself as insecure. Sometimes insecurity leads a person to be arrogant or even aggressive. In Tamika's case, it was plainly a lack of self-confidence. As we talked, she identified a problem from her past that seemed to be at the root of her current problem. It appeared that she grew up with an insecure internal working model. Her love cup was in deficit. Through her entire adolescence and up to the present, Tamika had grown up with her parents making comments comparing her to other girls her age. From the size of breasts, to athletic ability, to boyfriend, to grades, and the list continued.

Whenever I come across a client with "hundreds of small ts," I'll ask them for one small t that is representative of their problems. In Tamika's case, her memory was one that represented a series of comparisons communicated by her parents. As a result, Tamika has had significant difficulty with self-confidence, being secure with who she is, and avoiding social comparisons in every area of her life.

> *Everybody is a genius. But if you judge a fish by its ability to climb a tree, it will live its whole life believing that it is stupid.*
>
> Albert Einstein

One of the effects of insecurity is a lack of self-acceptance. The solution is coming to a place of loving oneself. This is different than self-focus and selfishness which impair relationships. Self-love and accepting yourself frees you up for authentic relating. Tamika began to find meaning in loving herself.

OVERCOMING INSECURITY WITH LOVE AND FORGIVENESS

I saw a 42-year old woman who grew up in Miami with a tough and hardened mother. Throughout childhood and adolescence she repeatedly heard: "You ain't gonna be nothing." It hurt for many years, but then she figured out that her mother was repeating what she had heard growing up. "I learned to ignore her, and then I learned to accept, forgive, and love her." And, after many years, she stopped saying the nasty things to me. "I once said to my mother, 'I figured out that you said those nasty things to me because that is what you were told for many years. But, I learned to ignore it. I made a decision a long time ago to forgive you and love you.' After that, my mother stopped saying those negative things."

Adversity can "break down" some people, but help others to become resilient. This woman is an example of a person who overcame a lifetime of insecurity and became resilient. And her love and forgiveness continues to bring healing to her mother.

INCONSISTENCY IMPAIRS RELATIONSHIPS

Inconsistency is not just an issue for individuals with bipolar disorder. If you take a deep interest in the lives of people, very often you will find inconsistency. Consider the father whose son needs consistent attention but doesn't get it; the child holds his father in high regard but the father is often distant and aloof. In this example, the child may experience intermittent attention,

> *Relationships are not a destination to be reached, but rather, a process to be lived.*
>
> John R. Buri

usually when the father is stress-free, has just achieved something and is happy, or it is holiday or vacation time. The problem is that these experiences are infrequent, and the child experiences inconsistent relating. The reasons for this father's parenting may be due to a number of factors including the legitimate stress of the economy. One of the HURTS involved may be the father's experience of his own father's inconsistency. Regardless, his inconsistency is providing a new HURT for his son.

Inconsistency in relating is seen in a number of relationship dynamics: bosses and supervisors, marriages and intimate partnerships, sibling relationships, and even customer service. As a result, people make the fundamental attribution error (Ross, 1977). Rather than saying, "Fred is having a bad day" or "Fred's work environment seems really stressful these days," people say, "Fred is a jerk!" But the inconsistency I'm referencing as an emotional consequence of some level of HURT is beyond rainy days, grumpy mornings, and seasonal trials. Very often, the problematic level of inconsistency is deeply rooted.

The solution is consistency in relationships. But, obtaining a set level of consistency is more a journey than a destination. It is something that you strive for with tomorrow as another opportunity to try to be consistent. Therapists can take time to discuss consistency at all levels of relationships with clients—both how they experienced or currently experience inconsistency from others and their own level of consistency in how they relate.

CYNICISM IMPAIRS RELATIONSHIPS

Some people use sarcasm regularly. In moderation, it can be humorous. Cynicism is a different way of relating. Cynicism is associated with pessimism, which is traditionally correlated with depression, hopelessness, and interpersonal problems. Recent research shows that optimists are better at regulating stress while pessimists were significantly less able to regulate their stress response and lower their cortisol levels over a 6-year period (Jobin, Wrosch, & Scheier, 2013). Poor stress management skills and increased cortisol levels affect interpersonal effectiveness.

A central aspect of pessimism is a person believing bad events will endure, will affect everything in life, and are completely their fault. When optimists face the same difficulties, they are resilient and unfazed by problems. They seem to get stronger in response to challenges. Optimists believe defeats are temporary obstacles and confined to one area of life; they also perceive bad or undesired situations as challenges that require increased effort (Seligman, 1991, 1996, 2002).

Pessimists are more likely going to give up. Thus, cynics or pessimists are likely going to lack effort in relationships or give up on them when things get a little difficult. When HURTS happen and remain unresolved, cynicism, or bitterness, often settles in. When people come out from the walls they are hiding behind, their communication with others is cynical rather than life-giving. Very often, therapy takes on the life of problem solving and helping the client to see the positive – finding the pearl in the dumpster. Sometimes therapy gains ground when the emphasis is placed on deeper levels of perspective.

DISAGREEABLENESS IMPAIRS RELATIONSHIPS

Some people with unresolved HURTS have a hard time saying what they think without leaving a bad impression, a bad taste, or a negative perception in others. Marketers, managers, and negotiators tend to be pros at making alternative points without others knowing that a disagreement is happening. Instead, it is happening in the flow of discovering truth, problem-solving, group flow, and the classic stages of forming, storming, norming, and performing (Tuckman, 1965).

Some people go through periods of time when they are spewing lemon juice. Rather than exerting a positive influence, they give off unpleasant aura. They can be disagreeable about anything or everything, and many other things get thrown into the mix. Instead of a good-natured disagreement, the disagreeableness is relationally difficult. Experienced therapists often see clients whose emotional entanglements result from an emphasis on divisiveness and disagreement. Therapists can take time to discuss how clients come across to others, regulate their emotion, increase empathy and disagree without being disagreeable.

HEALING FROM SMALL TS

Healing from small ts occurs in a 5-step process: (1) Therapists help clients identify small ts that are influencing current problems; (2) If necessary, therapists help clients separate small ts and big Ts; (3) For those clients who need a breakthrough, therapists incorporate a small t examination of emotional history to identify underlying small t's that are producing emotional entanglements; (4) Therapist and client collaboratively identify behavior that may be occurring in response to the small ts; (5) Collaboratively, therapist and client begin to identify alternative beliefs and behavior.

The goal of the small t examination of emotional history is to identify the origin of emotional responses. Therapist and client take a trip down memory lane together to identify specific small t memories that may be the origin of current emotional entanglements.

Sometimes this last step may involve writing a new narrative together. What was previously called a maladaptive personal story line (Binder & Betan, 2013), can now be established as a new narrative with different actions aimed towards more fulfilling and healthier relationships. Helping a client create a new story about his or her life involves questioning past faulty assumptions, a willingness to draw a line in the sand to declare openness to change, receptivity to modifying core attitudes, and establishing new approaches to work and relationships.

TRAUMA THERAPY INVOLVES A POSITIVE ASSET SEARCH

Trauma healing requires a search for positive assets. For therapists helping someone recover from a traumatization, there are questions that can draw out strengths and remind the client that growth can follow adversity and positives can be drawn from negatives. Such questions include:

- Have you had a change in your outlook?
- Do you value your relationships much more now?
- Are you more understanding and tolerant of others?
- Do you value other people more now?
- Are you able to perceive benefit in some areas in your life that you didn't before? For example, has this traumatic event taught you that you can handle anything? Or, because of what you have been through, are you more sensitive to the needs of others? Have you come to a place of seeing how good people can be based on those who have been there to help and support you?
- Do you have a sense of being able to thrive under pressure more effectively?
- Have you learned that you are stronger than you thought you were?
- Are you a more optimistic person?
- Have you become more grateful?
- Are you more appreciative of your friends and family?

- Are you more appreciative of life?
- Are you more appreciative of God?
- Do you have more empathy for others given what you have been through?
- Are you a more patient person and less likely to react to the small things of life?
- Are you able to identify growth following your adversity?
- Do you have more clarity about the priorities in your life?
- Do you have more appreciation for the value of your own life?
- Do you have greater optimism?
- Do you have deeper faith and or a stronger religious commitment?
- Have you increased your hopefulness as a result of what you have been through?
- Have you developed the "if I can get through that, I can get through anything" type of attitude?

IF YOUR ANSWER IS "NO" TO ALL THESE QUESTIONS

If answers to all of these questions is "no," this client is not alone. It is hard to come to this place after surviving a trauma. Healing takes time. Clients may not have more appreciation for the value of their life yet, but people tend to feel better when they look for ways to find gratitude and reduce the amount of bitterness.

COUNT YOUR BLESSINGS

In a classic study, Robert Emmons and Michael McCullough (2003) randomly assigned participants to one of three experimental conditions. One group would make a list of hassles: "hard-to-find parking," "financial problems," and "stupid people driving." Another group would make a list of neutral activities such as "talked to a colleague" or "cleaned out my shoe closet." The third group generated examples of experiences for which they were thankful such as "the generosity of friends," "to God for giving me determination," "for wonderful parents." The groups would regularly review these lists for 10 weeks. This study and subsequent research reveals the truth about gratitude that resembles age-old wisdom. Those who count their blessings each night are going to be happier. And, gratitude is the big buffer turning trauma into growth.

THE 2ND TYPE OF TRAUMA IS THE BIG T

Some small ts become laughable and embarrassing moments. When I was in the 7th grade, Leon and Jose saw me picking my nose during a filmstrip and to my distress and embarrassment nicknamed me Digger. In recent years, I found Leon on Facebook and reminded him of the incident. He humorously replied, "Yeah, we were cruel juveniles, but you were digging!"

Many small ts influence and impair us emotionally and lead to thought patterns like insecurity. While a small t is: "You'll never be able to hold a job" or: "You are an ugly girl," the Big T is influential not just on personality and belief dimensions but also produces distressing memories and anxiety symptoms. A big T is a parent being physically abusive and hitting repeatedly. Beliefs that result include: "I'm a horror," "I'm unlovable," and "I'm not good enough."

> *Resilience is not a commodity you are born with, waiting silently on tap. It is self-manufactured painstakingly over time by working through your problems and never giving up, even in the face of difficulty or failure.*
>
> Lorii Myers

And, sometimes big Ts are obviously <u>Traumatic</u>. In Southwest Florida, a woman came in for therapy after cleaning up brain parts after her mother's boyfriend shot himself in her mother's bedroom, because she and her mother couldn't afford the two grand for a professional clean-up company. In the Tampa area, a man swimming in a river experienced a lightning strike that left a hole in the back of his head; he regularly experiences intrusive recollections and flashbacks whenever he feels water hit his head from a shower and he has been avoiding swimming since the 2007 incident. A woman was left on a railroad track after being shot three times, with one bullet going through her eye ball; she survived and came in for treatment with her hair covering her missing eyeball. Or, a man who was attacked by a dog and had deep scars that looked like railroad tracks.

SMALL ts VERSUS BIG Ts CAN DEPEND ON RISK FACTORS

In the process of assessment, why do some people develop PTSD and others do not? I saw a professional and family woman who, while driving, had hit and killed someone. She served eight years for manslaughter, but didn't develop PTSD. Another woman had a simple accident and avoided driving for years. The difference between these women is difficult to explain.

There are some risk factors that influence the small versus big T distinction. First, prior anxiety disorders or substance abuse disorders are risk factors for the development of PTSD (Breslau et al., 1998). Lower intellectual functioning is a risk factor for the development of PTSD (Macklin et al., 1998). The prevalence of PTSD in twins indicates that 30% of some PTSD symptoms such as re-experiencing symptoms, avoidance of stimuli related to the trauma, and increased arousal are genetic (True et al., 1993). Another genetic risk factor is family history; trauma survivors with PTSD were more likely to have parents with mood problems, anxiety disorders, and substance abuse problems (Davidson et al., 1985).

There are neurobiological risk factors for PTSD. One is the reduction in hippocampal volume associated with PTSD which inhibits the hypothalamic-pituitary-adrenal axis, the body's stress response system (Bremner, Elzinga, Schmahl, & Vermetten, 2008). Another risk factor that has been identified is a genetic tendency toward exaggerated amygdala reactivity (Hariri et al, 2002). Personality traits such as neuroticism, is another risk factor of PTSD (Lesch et al, 1996). Low cortisol levels at the time of exposure to psychological trauma may also influence the impact of the traumatization (Resnick, Yehuda, Pitman, & Foy, 1995).

The question about why one person develops PTSD and another with more significant trauma does not, is sometimes explained by the aforementioned risk factors, but not always. Unfortunately, this professional conversation on theory and study goes well beyond the reach of this book. At the end of the day, it is the job of the therapist to help a client differentiate small from big Ts in therapy.

BIG TS ARE RELATIONAL

If a parent falls down the stairs after tripping over some toys, a broken arm may be traumatic to a mild degree. Often, this story becomes a memorable story in the journey of life (e.g., "I had stitches here;" "check out this mark where I fell off the rock"). If it remains a distressing memory, it is usually a small t (if at all) primarily because it is not relational. Sure, as a parent with a broken arm after tripping over a toy and falling down the stairs, we may blame a child momentarily or even blame ourselves because we were rushing and didn't follow the regular pre-bed routine of (1) clean

> *Great hearts can only be made by great troubles. The spade of trouble digs the reservoir of comfort deeper, and makes more room for consolation.*
>
> Charles Spurgeon

up our toys, (2) brush our teeth, (3) read three books, (4) say our blessings, etc. But, the bottom line is Big Ts occur when your spouse or father pushes you down the stairs. Non-relational accidents require exposure to actual or threatened death or serious injury.

NORMALIZING DISSOCIATIVE REACTIONS

I've been an advisory board member and an expert contributor on post-traumatic stress disorder for a wonderful organization called Selah Freedom in Sarasota, Florida. Selah Freedom is working to confront the issue of sexual trauma and exploitation through prevention and restoration services for survivors of sex trafficking. I've talked with many mental health clinicians who have had no (zero) conversations in any of their classes in graduate school on the realities of sex trafficking. Graduate students learn about psychological testing, abnormal psychology, research methods and other important topics to prepare for the licensure and practice of psychology, but not this horrific reality.

Recent studies estimate that approximately 18,000 to 50,000 people are trafficked into the United States annually. Florida is one of the top three "destination states" for trafficking. They are trafficked for forced labor (agriculture industry), domestic servitude (nail salons, hotel industry) or the sex industry. And, contrary to judgments, these girls and women are not "making a bad choice;" most are forced into the sex industry. I'd like to see graduate training in social work, counseling, and psychology increase their education on the assessment and treatment of survivors of modern-day slavery. This large topic is beyond the scope of what can be covered here, but additional resources (such as the U.S. Dept. of State Diplomacy In Action) and sources to educate yourself about human trafficking are included in the back of this book.

The critical and relevant factor for clinicians is providing treatment for survivors of sex trafficking and others who have experienced prolonged and chronic trauma. Victims often live in a perpetual state of fear and chronic anxiety. The body is classically conditioned to be in a state of hypersensitivity and hypervigilance. One of the more common problems in these complex cases is dissociative reactions that intrusively emerge. They often feel like "attacks on the consciousness" and anxiety about these

> *In order to succeed, people need a sense of self-efficacy to struggle together with resilience to meet the inevitable obstacles and inequities of life.*
>
> Albert Bandura

symptoms elevates. The normal two-step process in anxiety disorders, anxiety about anxiety (i.e. fear of having a panic attack), takes on a three-step process with complex trauma. The three-step process is actually anxiety about anxiety about dissociative reactions. Normalizing these symptoms and experiences for clients is step 1 for fostering freedom.

> *Resilience is accepting your new reality, even if it's less good than the one you had before.*
>
> Elizabeth Edwards

Dissociation Develops Into a 3-Step Spiral

Dissociative reactions, such as flashbacks in which the individual feels or acts as if the traumatic event were recurring, often happen spontaneously or in response to a trigger (e.g., opening or slamming of a door). Such reactions occur on a continuum with the most severe expression being a complete loss of awareness of present surroundings. Sometimes, a trafficking victim, now free and in recovery, may feel like she is back in the trapped room; being triggered toward feelings of unreality and the past is normal for this person. Coming back to the present, even when prompted by family members, may take time.

Typical responses following trauma are usually called sympathetic reactions, or more commonly described as flight or fight responses. Flight, fight, or freeze responses (frozen in fear) occur as a response to danger or perceived danger. Following trauma, danger is perceived more often. When the perceived danger exceeds the individual's ability to tolerate the emotional pain, dissociation is experienced.

It is common for complex and chronic trauma to involve depersonalization or derealization. Depersonalization involves the persistent experience of feeling detached from one's thoughts or body. A survivor may

> *Human beings have enormous resilience.*
>
> Muhammad Yunus

feel like she is in a dream or may feel like time is in slow motion. Derealization involves the persistent or recurrent experiences of surroundings seeming unreal. For example, it is common for a survivor's current bedroom to feel like it is not real; rather her "past room when I was tied up" seems to be reality at present. When Lisa experiences derealization, her present and safe room may seem distant, distorted (e.g., why aren't there bars on the windows?), or dreamlike.

The three-step process involves anxiety symptoms like heart palpitations, chest pressure, and nausea that follow dissociation. Consequently, these symptoms occur in anticipation of dissociation. It's not just worry about panicking or having flashbacks, it is now (1) anxiety and worry about (2) the "sick feelings:" chest pressure, heart palpitations, psychological and physiological distress with feelings of dread about what happened that leads to (3) dissociative symptoms. Dissociation involves anxiety about anxiety leading to dissociation. Nervousness and worry about having anxiety symptoms leads to increased dissociative feelings. Being paralyzed by fear is common for abuse survivors.

THE POWER OF VISUAL IMAGE REPLACEMENT

At this point, let's transition to treatment modalities for each of the facets of complex traumatization. Each of the symptoms of chronic post-traumatic stress disorder has a matching remedy. Below is a 20 for 20 table, 20 remedies for each of the 20 PTSD symptoms identified in the DSM-5®.

One of the key remedies is visual image replacement. This involves identifying a "safe place" and visualizing that place with all its colors, textures, sounds, and smells. Details of the image are elaborated in great detail. The safe place can match a picture on the client's wall or a picture of a place he or she has been to. When trust is built, a therapist can ask a client to describe out loud and in detail the visual aspects of the place. When therapists guide clients with visual imagery, the client is invited to close their eyes and identify a place of peace, relaxation, and safety.

When I worked with Jenny, she was a sexual assault survivor and demonstrated incredible courage just to come in for therapy. Jenny's story was an experience of being raped by a dentist on a military base. Prior to the rape, she had received inferior alveolar nerve anesthesia for the lower teeth and jaw. The injection blocked sensation in the inferior alveolar nerve, which runs from the angle of the mandible down the medial aspect of the mandible, innervating the lower teeth, lower lip, chin, and tongue. She was unable to yell during the incident and, with great fear and trepidation due to threat, understandably was unwilling to report the assault. I saw her a couple of years later, and her flashbacks

> *I am extremely interested in how people negotiate catastrophe, not because I'm morbidly interested in it but because I'm interested in the secret of resilience; that's what I'm always exploring in the stories and the novels.*
>
> Janette Turner Hospital

> *Life is ten percent what happens to you and ninety percent how you respond to it.*
>
> Lou Holtz

were intense. Her "safe place" that she used for visual image replacement was sitting on a beach watching a sunset. After practicing progressive relaxation (tense for five seconds and release of each of the major muscle groups) and practicing diaphragmatic breathing, she elaborated on the colors and beauty of her safe place. This location was a place she had gone to when she made tough decisions in the past, so it was associated with emotional muscle. It represented strength in her background so the image wasn't going to disintegrate under a tidal wave of excruciating images and emotional pain. This visual image was her source of image replacement when she experienced intrusive images and flashbacks about her traumatic memory.

20 Remedies for 20 Symptoms

1) Intrusive recollections	1) Thought replacement
2) Distressing dream	2) Reality check
3) Dissociative reactions such as a flashback	3) Visual image replacement
4) Increased distress at exposure to cue (sunglasses)	4) Thought about tolerating anxiety
5) Physical reaction (HR)	5) Thought about tolerating anxiety
6) Avoid thoughts, feelings, and conversations	6) Exposure when ready
7) Avoid activities, places or people that remind	7) Exposure when ready
8) Can't remember aspects of trauma	8) Acceptance
9) Diminished interest	9) Do it even if you don't feel like it.
10) Feeling detached	10) Work on a relationship by showing interest and asking another a question
11) Persistent and distorted blame of self or others	11) Letting-go intervention
12) Persistent negative emotional state (horror, guilt, or shame)	12) Gratitude exercises – Count 3 blessings each night and why did the blessing happen
13) Reckless or destructive behavior	13) Mindfulness and flow strategy to stop the urges
14) Restricted range of affect	14) Help another person

(Continued)

15) Foreshortened future	15) Plan out your vision for your future (even if you don't feel like it)
16) Difficulty with sleep	16) Deep breathing and apply insomnia-reversing strategies later in this book
17) Anger	17) Applied tension – relaxation
18) Difficulty concentrating	18) Say "in" for 3 seconds, then "out" for 3 seconds
19) Hypervigilance	19) Reality check and deep breathing
20) Exaggerated startle response	20) Accept, breathe, and tolerate

THE POWER OF MINDFULNESS

Mindfulness is a psychological quality that involves bringing one's complete attention to the present experience, being fully immersed in the moment by purposely paying attention to the present moment. Mindfulness is strongly related to acceptance of physiological sensations, no matter how uncomfortable. Much of what is in this book is about changing the whispering in one's interior life–those quiet thoughts that nag and aggravate. One of the roads to change is acceptance.

> *Always looking to the horizon. Never his mind on what he was doing.*
>
> Yoda

When I worked at the Hazelden Fellowship Club, a dual treatment program in St. Paul, Minnesota, I came to realize that the serenity prayer was powerful for recovering addicts coming to a place of letting go and acceptance. *God grant me the serenity to accept the things I cannot change; courage to change the things I can and wisdom to know the difference.* I have a friend named Fred, a recovering alcoholic, who I attended college with. We had a lot in common including talking lots about basketball. He often referenced the serenity prayer whenever he referenced his determination about staying sober.

At the heart of mindfulness is acceptance. And, acceptance is different from determination. Both acceptance and determination are key parts of cognitive behavior therapy. Acceptance or mindfulness involves observing the feelings in your body and NOT reacting to them, just accepting them. Determination involves doing something even if you don't feel like it (e.g., going to therapy

> *Train yourself to let go of everything you fear to lose.*
>
> Yoda

even when anxiety goes up). Both have their place. Below are the Dos and Don'ts of mindfulness, which is largely about observing and accepting.

Do	Don't
Observe and notice the feelings and sensations in your body. Notice the location of these feelings.	Don't try to change the bodily sensations.
	Don't try to push the emotions away.
Mentally, tell yourself to accept the situation and accept your reaction to the situation and to these feelings in your body.	Don't wrestle to fight the frustration; let go.
	Don't try to push the thoughts out of your mind.
Like an outside observer, notice the thoughts going on in your mind. Observe the thoughts like you're watching a train go by.	Don't try to make the discomfort go away.
	Don't reject your feelings.
Accept these thoughts and your feelings.	

DISSOCIATION REQUIRES A COMBINATION OF REMEDIES

To offset dissociative reactions, a combination of remedies is required: (1) visual image replacement, (2) mindfulness, (3) strategies to establish flow, and (4) reality checks.

It is recommended that therapists hand out the 20 for 20 table to their patients. (See pp. 53–54) For those patients struggling with dissociation, these four remedies should be emphasized. Visual image replacement involves using guided imagery to establish safe images that can replace images encompassed in flashbacks. Mindfulness exercises help generate acceptance of feelings reducing the strain that often accompanies feelings of dread and fearfulness associated with depersonalization and derealization.

> *Show me someone who has done something worthwhile, and I'll show you someone who has overcome adversity.*
>
> Lou Holtz

The study of flow is rooted in positive psychology (Csíkszentmihály, 1997). Flow is essentially being immersed in the moment, one with the music. Consider the rock climber who doesn't worry about his bills because he is so engaged in the moment. Csíkszentmihály identified certain factors that are required for flow; some of them include clear, attainable, but challenging goals, and engaging in an activity that is intrinsically rewarding. When you are in flow, time seems to stop, because you are so focused on the present that you lose track of time and lose awareness of physical needs among other components of the experience. Examples of flow include playing chess, skiing, mastering a skill in school, engaging in challenging athletic activities, or working on challenging work projects.

REALITY CHECKS ARE A CENTRAL TRAUMA REMEDY

A central feature of PTSD and trauma-based disorders is: "It's happening again." Accordingly, the essential treatment remedy is to come to a place of being able to say that it's not happening again. For Jose, an Iraq war veteran with immense anxiety about losing brothers in a set of road-side bombing ambushes, his symptoms elicited fear that he is re-experiencing the trauma. When he awakens from the nightmare, doing a reality check helps him identify that it's not 2004 anymore, he's not used to Iraq sand on his dinner plate, and he is living in St. Petersburg, Florida.

Reality checks involve a series of questions: Where am I? What is the date? What am I doing today? Who am I going to see? What am I going to eat? What time am I going to exercise? Who in my family am I going to text? When am I going to spend 20 minutes on Facebook® today? Are there two friends that I can call today?

One of the goals of reality checks involves having clarity about what is in the past. It's not Vietnam anymore. I don't live in that old apartment. I'm not living with the abusive uncle anymore. It's not happening again; the assault was 12 years ago. I'm not in that marriage anymore. I'm not in danger anymore.

Visual image replacement, mindfulness, strategies to establish flow, and reality checks are not easy to remember when anxiety heightens and dissociative reactions are triggered. Therapeutic reminders on this combination of remedies help greatly – How are you doing integrating these strategies? How has it been going? "Let's take 5 minutes at the onset here to discuss how visual image replacement, mindfulness, increasing flow strategies, and reality checks have been going. I have a lot of compassion for you and I realize it is not easy."

THE R2D2 HOLOGRAM AND TRAUMA THERAPY

There is a part in *Star Wars IV: A New Hope*, when R2D2 shows a hologram of Princess Leia to Obi Wan Kenobi. "Help me Obi Wan Kenobi, you're my only hope. Help me Obi Wan Kenobi, you're my only hope." There is a metaphor in this memorable movie moment as it relates to trauma survivors.

Consider light that exudes from you as the joy and freedom you experience. The hologram like the one R2D2 exuded represents the light in you. Thus, the brighter the light, the more joy and freedom experienced. The dimmer the light, the less joy and freedom experienced. As people get together with their loved ones, the hologram becomes brighter. As people avoid others, which is common for trauma survivors, the dimmer the hologram. This metaphor is a powerful tool to help nip at the heels of the avoidance issue following trauma. The brighter the hologram, the happier and healthier the person.

Beyond Symptom and Avoidance Reduction

The goal of trauma therapy is to help clients and patients to have a brighter hologram. Getting at the root of the trauma problem involves bringing traumatic memories to resolution. These unresolved memories are those memories that are stuck in the brain until they are processed. Unresolved or unprocessed memories keep emotions, beliefs, and physiological sensations trapped as they were experienced at the time of the traumatic event. Resolution involves getting the emotions up and out, processing through the traumatic verbal and emotional material, and assigning meaning to the experience.

The goal of trauma therapy is to process through unresolved memories and become unafraid of memories by reducing the anxiety associated with these memories. Assessing readiness is a key element of trauma therapy. An operational definition of readiness is a healthy balance of external support resources and internal coping resources. Severe depression, acute psychosis, suicide ideation, and active substance abuse are examples of deficient resources and would make trauma therapy beyond symptom and avoidance reduction contraindicated. Upon readiness, guiding therapy into exposure of the trauma memory requires an awareness of time, the client's motivation level, and the therapeutic zone. The deeper level of therapy of the therapeutic zone is the next step beyond symptom and avoidance reduction.

Thinking About the Therapeutic Zone

Let's pause and consider a basketball analogy in terms of getting into "the zone." More and more, basketball decisions are being made based on statistics and probability. Statisticians using advanced analytics analyze every movement and statistic. This includes spatial and visual analytics assessing frequency - which players shoot the most at different spots. As a simple example, if the ball can't get inside for an easy two (i.e. dunk/ lay-up), then 3-pointers are more likely. Over

> *Life is about timing.*
>
> Carl Lewis

the years at the highest levels, more 3-point attempts are being taken on average per year. Consider these simple statistics: Players shooting 30% of 50 3-pointers results in 45 points; players shooting 42% of 50 2-point shots results in 42 points. Consequently, coaches disfavor long two-point shots and manage the offensive sets around being "close to the basket" or "beyond the arc." Games are managed based on strategy and getting a team into a zone of maximizing probability.

This basketball analogy has some relevance. The therapeutic zone is not based on probability but there are similarities between the job of a basketball coach and the job of a therapist—such as getting into the right zone. There are many aspects of the client's care to manage when approaching trauma exposure. Of course, assessing readiness is a prerequisite. In some ways, the process is simple – facilitate a respectful and caring environment where a person can talk about a traumatic event. In other ways, it is complex, and awareness of the therapeutic zone is helpful.

ENTERING THE THERAPEUTIC ZONE

Like strategy coaching in basketball, the therapist is mindful of many factors in therapy. One of the things that helps to balance is drawing out thoughts versus drawing out feelings. Metaphorically, the zone involves working the ball towards the basket and balancing cognitive and emotion questions. At the start of the session, initial emotional arousal is common for clients much like pre-game performance arousal for athletes. After warm up chit-chat and rapport building (catching up on the week), the emotional arousal sometimes subsides. In these situations, the client may start to become comfortable with therapy again.

Trauma therapy then consists of bringing clients into the therapeutic zone. At approximately one quarter of the way into the session (at the 25% mark), the therapist carefully elevates the level of emotional activation the client experiences. The goal here is to help the client begin to experience a level of intense emotion that he or she can tolerate. The goal is to get into the center of the therapeutic zone. Going too far beyond the zone may cause the client to be flooded with emotion beyond their coping ability or their capacity to regulate the traumatic emotion. Too little activation keeps the session in supportive therapy, which is sometimes what the client needs. These times are opportunities for strength building and positive asset searches. But, trauma therapy involves bringing the client to the zone by elevating the intensity of the therapy experience allowing the client to learn to tolerate the traumatic material. With one fourth of the session time remaining (at the 75% mark), the therapist should work to reduce the level of emotional activation. For the client's emotional safety, as the session nears its conclusion, his or her level of arousal should be lower than when he or she came into the office.

After processing and the client's arousal is lowered, some metaphors are helpful. Remind clients that they might experience reminders (i.e. images) of what was just discussed spontaneously throughout the week. This experience is normal. If it happens, allowing it, accepting it, and letting it flow past is helpful. Also, deciding at the end of the session to put the cap back on the bottle sends the message that the client is in charge of taking the cap off. And, when they do, to do it slowly. This does two things – reinforces an internal locus of control and reminds them to go at things slowly.

INFLUENCING THE THERAPEUTIC ZONE

Therapists influence clients in the therapeutic zone by increasing or decreasing the level of emotion activation in session. The purpose of this emotional activation is sometimes negatively interpreted as "reliving the trauma." In actuality, the purpose is to douse the associations connected to the trauma. Trauma therapy involves activating and then healing. During the following process, sometimes interpreting defenses such as describing the trauma without affect is needed. Additionally, alliance-building comments, "I'm right here with you" and "you aren't alone here" can help with feelings of vulnerability.

Trauma processing starts with encouraging the client to take some deep breaths and relax as much as possible. The client is asked to close his or her eyes and describe the traumatic memory slowly with as much detail as can be remembered. Encourage the client to use present-tense language. Examples include "he is entering the bedroom" versus "he entered the bedroom." Arouse the senses by asking the client to expand on sensory details: sounds she or he is hearing, what colors and images look like, smells, tastes (if appropriate such as dry mouth during fear elevation), or thoughts going through his or her mind. The telling of the story in the present tense brings the client to the moment of exposure (in a safe and therapeutic situation) to the traumatic memories of the past. The therapist gently encourages the story-telling. The center of the zone is inviting the client to explicitly identify the most distressing moment of the trauma.

Questions that raise the arousal level are emotion questions such as sensory details. General emotion questions include: "Could you tell me more about that?" "What was that like?" The most brief and straight-forward question is: "What else?" Repeatedly asking "what else?" is sometimes enough to bring out the experience. The goal is asking questions that draw out the emotion and experience.

QUESTIONS TO REDUCE AROUSAL

Cognitive questions are those primarily intended to reduce arousal. Some increase arousal such as those negative beliefs about self like: "I am a horror." Distancing and changing these negative beliefs are a part of therapy. Timing is important for work in the therapeutic zone. Arousal is reduced due to session time or to help the client not exceed the therapeutic zone and become flooded ("I need a break" or "this is too much"). Again, reducing arousal is needed at approximately the 75% mark of the session.

The following are thought questions that help reduce arousal, increase distance from the emotional trauma, and begin to re-establish the present as distinct from the past. This is critical to the idea that, "it's not happening again." "It's not happening now."

Here are some examples of thought questions: "Why do you think someone might do that?" "What do you think goes through a person's mind for them to do something like that?" "What do you think you would tell your friend about her step-father, had this happened to her?" Sometimes direct communication is needed to help transition: "At this point, let's begin to push pause on the processing." "But there is something I am wondering about, what do you think...?" The goal is to access some logic or critical (or uncritical) thinking. We want to decrease amygdala activation and increase frontal lobe activity which involves thinking, learning, abstracting, inhibiting, and reasoning.

STRENGTH BUILDING AND REFLECTION

The following session may involve continued trauma processing. One of the essential things to do after any part of trauma reprocessing is strength building. The following strengths are based on the Values In Action (VIA) Classification of Character Strengths (Peterson & Seligman, 2004) and some in particular are poignant strengths for trauma healing such as *courage*. Other strengths include *bravery* (*valor*) which involves not withdrawing from threat, challenges, or pain. *Creativity* is relevant for thinking of novel and productive ways to solve problems. *Perseverance* is a critical strength in therapy and looking for three ways the client perseveres is strength-building. Facilitating an opportunity for the client to talk about what the processing was like is important. And, reflection time is an excellent opportunity to honor the client for his or her strengths.

Other strengths are helpful to build upon in various aspects of cognitive behavioral therapy: Curiosity, judgment (critical thinking), love of learning, perspective (wisdom), integrity and honesty, zest, love, kindness, social intelligence, teamwork, fairness, leadership, forgiveness, humility, self-regulation, appreciation of beauty and excellence, gratitude, humor, and faith and purpose. Research indicates that encouraging clients to deploy their highest strengths increases flow–fully engaged activity involving the experience of being one with the music (Seligman, 2011). Identifying activities (and perhaps a new hobby) is also a great way to redirect toward something outside of therapy in which the client can use these strengths. For reliable and valid questionnaires to measure strengths and other positive qualities like grit, optimism, gratitude, happiness, and meaning, see the website www.authentichappiness.org.

> *Change is not made without inconvenience, even from worse to better.*
>
> Richard Hooker

Below is a list of positive psychology interventions that therapists use to supplement cognitive-behavioral interventions. These are particularly instrumental in supplementing healing work in trauma therapy.

Positive Psychology Intervention	Goal
Identify top five strengths and find new ways to implement them	Increases flow
Identify personal difference maker and write a gratitude letter	Increases gratitude and happiness
Name five things you are grateful for – 30 Days	
Deliberately reminisce and savor good times (read old journals)	
Intentionally engage in acts of kindness (five a day)	Build memories
Establish new rituals (i.e. prayer, exercise, gratitude journal)	Increase selflessness
	Clarity on values/vision
See self as 105 years old, what advice would you give to your younger self.	Perspective broadening

I've recently worked with a 105-year old client. She said to me that her boyfriend, who is in his 80's is afraid of commitment, which adds much humor to life. There is nothing that broadens perspective like a 100+ year old talking about life issues.

CHAPTER 4

Building Anxiety Tolerance and Becoming Unafraid

BUILDING ANXIETY TOLERANCE TAKES SMALL STEPS

A generalized protocol for anxiety treatment involves (1) building anxiety tolerance, (2) avoidance reduction, and (3) reframing exaggerated threat appraisals. Building anxiety tolerance is like a therapist mining for gold, searching for admirable qualities in their clients. Those qualities are then drawn out as a way to prepare for the building of emotional muscle. This chapter focuses on how emotional muscle is built through building anxiety tolerance, by eliminating avoidance, and by noticing the exaggeration in appraising threats and beginning to appraise differently. This is largely emphasized with exposure and other behavioral experiments.

GOING TO THE MOVIES ALONE

I'm a big fan of going to the movies by yourself. But, sometimes anxiety reduction takes steps. Yes, the fear hierarchy is an oldie but a goodie. Oldies are often forgotten in newly packaged treatments that secure gold standard efficacy study evidence. It was Joseph Wolpe, once a dedicated follower of Freud who ended up leaving psychoanalytic therapy to search for

> *Courage does not always roar. Sometimes courage is the quiet voice at the end of the day saying, "I will try again tomorrow."*
>
> Mary Ann Radmacher

more efficacious treatments, who developed the reciprocal inhibition and systematic desensitization principles behind the anxiety hierarchy.

In working with Margaret, a client with social anxiety, it took four sessions just to establish that trust was an issue due to small ts from her family of origin. Basically, it was like pulling teeth. My behavioral observations of her in early sessions were that she was shy, timid, and withdrawn. But, she courageously kept returning to therapy. Most pressing was Margaret's anxiety in social situations. Assigning going to the movies alone was not a manageable homework assignment. We identified a list of anxiety-producing situations from least distressing to most distressing. Wolpe called the level of anxiety – subjective units of distress (SUDS).

We identified Margaret's fear hierarchy and developed a plan for her to approach each item one by one every other day. We practiced muscle relaxation developed by Edmund Jacobson in the early 1920's and updated by Bernstein & Borkovec (1973). This involved tensing one muscle group at a time. In my sessions with Margaret, we worked on two muscle groups per week (2 total minutes). In the process, Margaret (1) closed her eyes, (2) was encouraged to let go and relax, (3) was encouraged to notice the tension in the specific muscle group being tensed (for 10 seconds at a time), (4) was encouraged to allow her body to relax and to notice the difference between the relaxation and the tension.

LET THE ABDOMEN EXPAND, NOT THE CHEST

A lifetime skill worthy of 5 minutes of therapy time and one-minute follow up questions in later sessions is teaching clients and patients diaphragmatic breathing. Diaphragmatic, or belly breathing made a significant difference for Margaret long-term. This breathing exercise involves expanding the abdomen. It is common for people to expand the chest as they breathe, which tightens the shoulders increasing physiological stress. The goal of diaphragmatic breathing is to counter the shallow breathing that often accompanies anxiety disorders.

FROM LEAST ANXIETY TO MAXIMUM ANXIETY

Identifying the least anxiety-producing situations to the most anxiety-producing situations is a collaborative process. What situation would be most anxiety-producing for you? For Margaret, "making a speech" and "going to the movies alone" were tied at 100 on the SUDS scale. Of course, sitting at home was the least anxiety-producing situation. Margaret practiced muscle relaxation and intentionally and mindfully made an effort towards diaphragmatic breathing before each step. Then, she faced her anxiety with the mindset of gradually building up her anxiety tolerance from 0, no

> If there is no struggle, there is no progress.
>
> Frederick Douglass

anxiety to 100, maximum anxiety. Below is Margaret's exposure and anxiety hierarchy of anxiety-producing social situations. After 12 sessions, Margaret went to the movies alone!

Margaret's Exposure Hierarchy of Social Situations	Level of SUDS - 0: no anxiety to 100: maximum anxiety
Sitting at home	10
Going for a drive alone	15
Going for a walk around the neighborhood	25
Going for a walk in a park	35
Walking the strip mall near the grocery store	40
Going to the movies with her sister	55
Eat breakfast at The Broken Egg (Dick Vitale's favorite spot in Sarasota, FL)	60
Go shopping at the mall	65
Go shopping for groceries alone	75
Go to a work get-together with colleagues	85
Participate in a group or class	90
Make a speech / go to the movies alone	100

BUILDING ANXIETY TOLERANCE VIA EXPOSURE

Therapeutic exposure is empowering for people and sets them free of anxiety and fear of uncertainty. By planning out exposure, clients begin to add structure to their lives. Rather than the unpredicted triggers that can elicit anxiety, therapists help clients prepare, plan, and even predict their level of anxiety and triggers that elicit anxiety. The first step is simple education that the client's anxiety is going to go up. This is the beginning step for increasing anxiety tolerance.

The second step is identifying triggers that elicit anxiety and developing behavioral approaches when confronted with these triggers such as muscle relaxation and diaphragmatic breathing. When confronted with triggers, helpful cognitive approaches include scaling, soothing self-talk (i.e. "I can tolerate emotional discomfort."), and cognitive restructuring (i.e. "the trigger is inconvenient, but not horrible.").

DECIDING, NOT SLIDING

A third step on building anxiety tolerance is developing the skill of critically evaluating the threat, as opposed to sliding back into the pattern of exaggerating the threat. One of the more common cognitive distortions is emotional reasoning, believing it is true because it feels true. The worst part of the anxiety-producing situation feels true because of threat exaggeration.

Reducing threat *exaggeration* and increasing threat *evaluation* requires deciding, not sliding. Clients with anxiety tend to slide into exaggerating a threat. Clients with GAD exaggerate worries, clients with OCD exaggerate uncertainties, clients with trauma memories exaggerate triggers, clients with social anxiety exaggerate the possibilities of embarrassment, and clients with panic exaggerate frightening bodily sensations. Deciding to critically evaluate the threat tends to establish new patterns and empower the client.

Fourth, building anxiety tolerance requires clarity that an essential goal is to help clients eliminate reliance on escape and avoidance strategies. Therapeutic exposure ("when you're ready") is about confronting fears and taking control of your life. When I teach seminars on anxiety to therapists, it is inevitable that an audience member will wonder why they should help a client confront a particular source of anxiety if it doesn't affect their current functioning. My response is often something along the lines of, "therapists need to use their clinical judgment in collaboration with their clients to develop the therapy goals and treatment plan and proceed accordingly." In other words, it may not be necessary to confront a fear if it doesn't affect daily living. But, I always throw in a caveat. And, it involves the notion of believing that nothing outside of a person should have control over their life. Becoming unafraid of anxiety involves freedom from fear and freedom from anything that may have a hold of a person's life.

I have an old friend and colleague who once experienced some sickness while eating Spaghettios® and then spent years avoiding the food. When I do training at the facility where she works, I'll make the similar comment of getting free from and not letting anything control your life. And, I joke that, "this includes Spaghettios," to her chagrin. But, it raises an important issue of living a life free of external control, because that is what these anxiety-producing situations are–sources of external control.

SITUATIONAL EXPOSURE BUILDS MUSCLE

Building muscle involves micro-tearing of muscle fibers during training, known as microtrauma. This microtrauma in the muscle contributes to the soreness we feel after weight training exercise. It is the repair of these fibers that leads to muscle growth. Essentially, the process involves breaking down muscles in order to build them back up. This is where the old adage "no pain, no gain" hits home for people.

In vivo exposure involves directly approaching activities in different situations building a different kind of muscle – emotional muscle. I walked with one client with hypsiphobia (fear of height) to a bridge when he was ready and we scaled his anxiety every 20 feet. Another example is when therapists direct someone who fears public speaking (glossophobia) to give a speech to others. These situational exposures build emotional muscle by increasing anxiety gradually but without avoidance, which usually strengthens the fear response. Instead, the therapist helps the client break the patterns of avoidance and thus the fear response.

As muscles become adapted to the exercises, soreness tends to decrease. Anxiety tolerance works in a similar way. As individuals adapt to certain situations, anxiety tends to decrease. This is the goal for fear of heights or speaking anxiety.

THERAPISTS NEED TO ASSESS FOR INTERNAL RESOURCES

Therapists need to help clients identify internal resources or instill these strengths within clients. When exposure interventions are done with clients with minimal resources, clients are at risk for increased problems and psychopathology. Exposure should not be used if the client has poor impulse control, uncontrolled substance use disorder, psychosis, suicidal ideation, or engages in non-suicidal self-injurious behavior. Finally, clients should have their standard physical examinations by their primary care physicians to assess for any medical contraindications for engaging in exposure interventions.

As an example of a client who was unready–I recently saw a client in St. Petersburg, Florida who was being treated by a therapist with the use of Eye Movement Desensitization and Reprocessing (EMDR). EMDR is an evidence-based treatment efficacious for a variety of psychological problems, most notably for PTSD. A meta-analysis of 38 randomized controlled trials suggested that the first-line psychological treatment for PTSD should be cognitive behavioral therapy that is trauma-focused or EMDR (Bisson et al., 2007). So, let's name this client Jill. She had a multi-year cocaine history and remained a chronic user–she used the day before her appointment. She was a sexual assault survivor and clearly met criteria for PTSD. I was seeing her for psychological testing to help with her vocational rehabilitation and learned of her recent and ongoing treatment with a clinician who was using EMDR. I was flabbergasted.

I share this story as I often tell audiences that young clinicians often error on the side of, "Oh, a chance for me to use this new treatment" rather than using wisdom and sound clinical judgment. I have a colleague who uses the phrase "everything is a nail to a hammer" in this context. It is common for excited therapists to leave treatment seminars perceiving every client as a nail. EMDR protocol and exposure protocols encourage sobriety first with the development of a strong set of internal resources prior to using a treatment that will only elevate relapse probability. Dual treatment programs popularized in recent years should not include exposure-based therapies that make clients vulnerable until sufficient internal resources have been developed. The story exposure protocol from chapter one is only for sober individuals capable and ready to face their own trauma.

> *Only a fully trained Jedi Knight, with the Force as his ally, will conquer Vader and his emperor.*
>
> Yoda

Even Aaron Beck, the father of cognitive therapy, warned in his classic *Cognitive Therapy for Depression* (1979) that amateur therapists are susceptible to emphasizing technique at the expense of what a person actually needs.

MEDICATION SHOULD BE EXAMINED

Building anxiety tolerance requires an accurate assessment of medication therapy. First and foremost, medication only alleviates symptoms, but psychotherapy or psychological treatment is what cures anxiety disorders. Let's take a look at the different classes of medications including anti-depressant medications prescribed for anxiety disorders.

SSRIs

Medications such as Prozac, Paxil, Zoloft, Celexa, and Lexapro are selective serotonergic reuptake inhibitors (SSRIs). They work by regulating serotonin levels in the brain to elevate mood and reduce symptoms. Common side effects include nausea, nervousness, headaches, sexual dysfunction, dizziness, and weight gain. Physiological dependence is not usually an issue, but SSRI's need to be discontinued slowly.

Tricyclics

Tricyclics such as imipramine (Tofranil) for panic disorder and GAD and clomipramine (Anafranil) for OCD are older than SSRI's but still prescribed for anxiety disorders. Common side effects include dizziness, drowsiness, dry mouth and weight gain.

Beta-Blockers

Beta-blockers such as propranolol (Inderal) are used to treat heart problems. Sometimes they are prescribed to treat some of the physical symptoms of anxiety.

MAOIs

Monoamine oxidase inhibitors (MAOIs) such as phenelzine (Nardil) and tranylcypromine (Parnate) are the oldest class of antidepressant medications but have been commonly prescribed for anxiety disorders. I am starting to see these medications less and less in clinical practice, because of the problems and side effects associated with their use. And, as clinicians have known for many years, taking these meds with cheese, red wine, pain relievers like Advil, cold medications, and birth control pills cause interaction effects such as problematic increases in blood pressure.

Anti-Anxiety Medications

Buspirone (Buspar) is a newer medication used to treat GAD with possible side effects of nausea, dizziness, and headaches.

The "quick fix" society is epitomized by alprazolam (Xanax) medication for anxiety, an FDA-approved but controversial medication. Xanax is a high-potency benzodiazepine along with clonazepam (Klonopin) used for social phobia and GAD, and lorazepam (Ativan) used for panic disorder. If benzos are needed, clonazepam or Xanax XR are often prescribed as they act more slowly, have longer half-lives, and can manage anxiety with less potential for negative reinforcement and thereby less psychological dependence.

THE XANAX BANDAID PREVENTS ANXIETY TOLERANCE

I recently provided anxiety treatment for a 26-year old nurse, an intelligent, well-connected professional. She commented during the course of cognitive-behavioral therapy that she has six or seven friends with "mood and anxiety issues" who all take medications, but do not engage in personal therapy. This comment reminded me of some of the problems in mental health–from the mental health stigma (damaging views about psychological problems and therapy) to reliance on medication therapy at the expense of the TRUE CURE – psychological treatment!

This reliance on medication therapy is best captured in the prescribing of Xanax

> *We have bigger houses and smaller families; more conveniences but less time; we have more degrees, but less sense; more knowledge, but less judgment; more experts, but more problems; more medicine, but less wellness.*
>
> George Carlin

for panic disorder and other anxiety problems. Xanax is a controversial treatment because people become dependent and can develop tolerance (Moylan, Gjorlando, Nordfjærn, & Berk, 2012). Xanax sedates rapidly with 90% of peak effects occurring within the first half hour and full peak effects achieved within 1 ½ hours (Sheehan, Sheehan, & Raj, 2007). Consequently, the "quick fix" treatment method for panic is Xanax. Xanax has high potency, a rapid onset, and a short half-life, characteristics that likely account for its status as a drug of abuse (Substance Abuse and Mental Health Services Administration, 2010). The long-term outcome of benzodiazepine use for anxiety disorders, is beyond the scope of this section, but the lack of long-term evidence of benzo therapy and other psychiatric medications is expounded upon (and questioned) in Robert Whittaker's *Anatomy of an Epidemic* (2010).

Clearly, benzos are very effective in alleviating anxiety for the short term, but they result in an increase of anxiety long-term. First, Xanax interferes with exposures and other treatment methods that require clients to experience anxiety so they can build tolerance and notice the strategies they use to bring the

> *If you accept the expectations of others, especially negative ones, then you never will change the outcome.*
>
> Michael Jordan

anxiety down. *In other words, experiencing anxiety is good, and not to be avoided.* Second, these quick-acting medications are used as "safety behaviors" which prevent facing fear directly. Taking benzodiazepines is the #1 dysfunctional safety behavior that negatively reinforces anxiety. *The goal is to reduce safety behaviors.* Third, these clients most often attribute their progress to medication rather than to their personal work on facing anxiety, elevating anxiety-related issues in therapy. *This limits and deprives clients of an increase in self-efficacy.*

XANAX IS FOR THOSE WHOSE HEADS ARE BARELY ABOVE WATER

Many clients require psychiatric medication: legitimate cases of bipolar disorder, that small percentage of legitimate and severe cases of ADHD, psychotic disorders like schizophrenia, and severe unipolar emotional disorders like severe depression. A recent meta-analysis (of 48 randomized controlled trials and 6,674 participants) found that lithium reduces the risk of suicide and total deaths by more than 60% compared with placebo in both unipolar and bipolar depressive disorder (Cipriani, Hawton, Stockton & Geddes, 2013). Clients on therapists' case loads who require psychiatric medication also include those whose anxiety is so severe that they are unable to function, leave their house, or get dressed, shower, bathe and groom themselves. Xanax is for those individuals whose heads are barely above water.

These are clients who require medication to function; exposure treatments and anxiety tolerance-building exercises will not be in their treatment plan in the near future. When the time is right, following improved functioning, elevating the bar of success can be re-evaluated. This takes clinical judgment, consideration of risk and protective factors, and wisdom. And, in these situations, therapy emphasis should be placed on finding meaning, eating well, consistent exercise, and sleeping well and regularly.

Then, there are those clients with limited coping strategies who rely on psychotropic medication. I have a friend, a social worker, who jokes about nurses at a nursing facility who are quick with PRNs, "Oh no, a feeling, let's give them a Xanax." But, this summarizes the approach to many clients with limited internal resources and coping strategies who depend on medication therapy.

Imaginal Exposure Is Real

While in vivo exposure uses a direct approach with specific triggers, imaginal exposure involves working with patients to visualize and "imagine" situations that they are afraid of. This is particularly strength-building for confronting feared images, thoughts, and memories. Imaginal exposure includes story exposure identified earlier in this book.

Reminding clients that "your anxiety will go up" is an example of communicating expectations with clients. Although there is a perception that talking about future anxiety makes experiences more difficult, thinking about future anxiety and normalizing it can actually help set clients up for greater success.

Trauma therapy consists of imaginal exposure. Much of what we discussed in Chapter 3 on guiding clients toward the therapeutic zone is imaginal exposure. With imaginal exposure, you are asking clients to mentally confront a situation that they are afraid of. For those specific phobias and "present anxiety-producing situations," imaginal exposure is the first step prior to in vivo exposure (real life exposure) such as visualizing bees prior to visiting a bee farm. Recent research shows that prior to in vivo exposure, watching someone else safely interact with fear-inducing objects (e.g., spiders) can help to extinguish conditioned fear responses (Golkar, Selbing, Flygare, Ohman, & Olsson, 2013).

AND SOMETIMES, A GARBAGE SESSION IS NEEDED

One of my all time favorite therapy sessions is what I call the <u>garbage session</u>. When a client I am talking with has obsessions over cleanliness, it reminds me of the power of the garbage session. To illustrate, after preparing the client, I once emptied my entire garbage onto the floor all around our feet. And, it was nasty. I had used Kleenex, old banana peels, and other junk not yet collected. The goal was direct in vivo exposure toward disorder, messiness, and disarray. Upon the dumping of the mess, Mauri's anxiety shot through the roof. As the minutes went by, her anxiety began to decrease as her tolerance increased. Sessions later, she reported increased tolerance with things out of place in her apartment. Her growing tolerance began to free her up to focus on her schoolwork and communication with friends that was previously delayed due to obsessions and subsequent cleaning. And, she began to clean with more flexibility and significantly lower anxiety at random times.

INTEROCEPTIVE EXPOSURE BUILDS TOLERANCE

Practicing exposures consist of in vivo exposure (i.e. Paul driving again after an accident) and imaginal exposure (i.e. Shannon seeing herself arrive at home with the house on fire). The third exposure intervention is interoceptive exposure, widely used for panic disorder and PTSD. Here, patients confront anxiety-producing bodily sensations like heart palpitations and shortness of breath.

> *My father used to say that it's never too late to do anything you wanted to do. And he said, 'You never know what you can accomplish until you try.'*
>
> Michael Jordan

Interoceptive exposure is the repeated reproduction of, and exposure to, uncomfortable arousal-related bodily sensations. The purpose is a reduction in the client's fear of specific bodily cues through repeated exposure to them. In other words, the goal is to become unafraid of bodily sensations and anxious tension. One of the hallmarks of panic is being afraid of panic. Interoceptive exposure is about experiencing panic in a therapeutic environment in order to be unafraid of panic– ultimately reducing panic.

In preparation, a therapist will, in a safe environment, inquire of a client about their experience of panic sensations. Have you ever experienced a panic attack and not felt like you were going to lose control? Have you ever been anxious and then panicked but begun to realize that the bodily sensations were tolerable? The therapist may then invite the client to put her face against the wall with her back to the therapist. The experience of being an inch away from the wall for two minutes can induce a panic attack. See the chart below for other scenarios that can be used to induce a panic attack in this setting.

The client then processes the experience in a safe environment. How was it? Could you tolerate it? Can you view these bodily sensations as uncomfortable rather than catastrophic? Could you view yourself experiencing these uncomfortable bodily sensations and still feel like you are in control? These types of questions are helpful in reframing the experience and the processing provides experiential practice of self-appraisals that will help in future panic incidents. Below is a list of interoceptive exposures and produced sensations.

Interoceptive Exposure	Produced Sensations
P90x© style push ups or simply jogging in place to increase HR; consider jumping jacks (oldie but goodie)	Racing heart, breathlessness, rapid breathing rate, chest pain and tightness
Hold nose and breathe through a straw for two minutes	Smothering sensations, "not getting enough air into lungs," pounding heart, choking, fear of suffocation
Spin around in a chair for 90 seconds	Dizziness or "fainting" feelings, accelerated or pounding heart, breathlessness, smothering sensations, nausea
"Like a kid" – see how long you can hold your breath. Try to reach for 30 seconds	Breathlessness, racing heart, dizziness
Face the wall with back to the therapist; stare at the same spot for 2 minutes	Feeling unreal, dizzy, and feelings of "being stared at"
Tense your muscles, much like progressive relaxation; start with one muscle group at a time or tense entire body	Trembling/shaking, breathlessness, pounding heart, smothering sensations

I first started using interoceptive exposures with a college student named Shelly. After she consented, Shelly stood with her nose one inch from the wall and stared at it until she started panicking. The intervention induced a panic attack. We then processed her ability to tolerate the symptoms. Upon reflection after the tenth session, Shelly pointed to the interoceptive exposure in session 4 as a highly memorable and beneficial experience.

These interventions only work if the therapist tailors the interoceptive exposure to the client's problems. It is the therapist's job to ensure that the feared symptoms are provoked and experienced. If the person fears nausea, then spinning around in a chair will directly provoke this symptom. Some clinicians have used low doses of Ipecac syrup as a way to induce nausea (Dattilio, 2003). A person with dental fears or claustrophobia may fear suffocation, as a result, breathing through a straw would be a precise intervention. Mckay & Moretz (2008) have used 3D glasses to induce depersonalization, common in patients with PTSD and panic disorder. The key is treatment matching. This, of course, requires a thorough assessment of feared symptoms. The goal is to become unafraid of these symptoms. "Oh, just like a headache, those are panic feelings."

Getting Back To Exercising

Clients with anxiety hypersensitivity and panic attacks tend to avoid exercise. While a common approach to stress is inactivity and cigarette smoking, a better approach is clean living and exercise. But comfort seeking due to low energy, anhedonia, other depression symptoms, or frankly laziness, only account for some of the variables that explain inactivity.

I had a patient named Lisa who avoided exercise because of "the way it makes me feel." When someone exercises, the heart rate accelerates, sweating increases, and other bodily sensations such as chest pressure remind people of what they dread–symptoms associated with a panic attack. The best interoceptive self-guided homework assignment is to get back to exercising. It is at the heart of Susan Jeffers' (1987) timeless classic *Feel the Fear and Do It Anyway*. This book is an important resource for clients who are conquering anxiety and one worth recommending. For Lisa, her "emotional breakthrough" occurred when she returned to her running and home fitness routine. "I avoided exercise because of the chest pressure, heart racing, and adrenaline pumping. But my breakthrough happened when I didn't view these symptoms negatively."

Helping clients establish or reestablish a regular exercise regimen following a relapse of panic is critical. In both cases, exercise helps patients gain more tolerance with bodily discomfort.

There Is Freedom in Avoidance Reduction

I mentioned at the beginning of this chapter that the generalized protocol for anxiety treatment involves (1) building anxiety tolerance, (2) avoidance reduction, and (3) reframing exaggerated threat appraisals.

The second part of becoming unafraid is avoidance reduction. This starts with a three-step process: (1) assessment of negative reinforcement in clients with anxiety disorders, (2) psycho-education on negative reinforcement, and, (3) establishing solution-oriented plans for each negatively reinforced behavior.

> *Change does not roll in on the wheels of inevitability, but comes through continuous struggle. And so we must straighten our backs and work for our freedom.*
>
> Martin Luther King, Jr.

LET'S ESTABLISH CLARITY ON NEGATIVE REINFORCEMENT

It is not uncommon for therapists and clients to be confused about negative reinforcement. So, let's establish clarity on negative reinforcement. Often, people think of a reward as positive reinforcement and a punishment as negative reinforcement. That is not the case! Let's take a moment to review the basics. In behavior modification, positive behavior is followed by positive consequences: positive and negative reinforcement. In contrast, undesired behavior should be followed by negative consequences, traditionally referred to as a punishment. In parenting, this may involve a timeout, a loss of a privilege, or a reprimand. Reinforcement mistakes occur when undesired behavior is reinforced. For example, a kid exhibits a tantrum when Mom says "No" and the mother changes her mind and gets him a candy to stop the tantrum. This parenting error reinforces poor emotional regulation skills, disobedience, poor listening, and many other behavior problems.

WHAT IS NEGATIVE REINFORCEMENT?

While positive reinforcement adds a "positive" to strengthen a behavior (i.e. wage increase following good performance), negative reinforcement is removing a "negative" or aversive stimulus that a person doesn't want leading to behavior that is "reinforced" or strengthened. Consider the following examples:

Negative Stimulus	Behavior That Is Reinforced
Insect bite itches	Scratch it
Lights too bright	Squint or shade eyes
Cold draft of air	Close the window
Too much nagging	Drown it out with the radio
Have a headache	Take a pain reliever

Psychologically, smoking has an anxiety reduction effect. When somebody is stressed and goes for a cigarette, the smoking reduces the prior experienced tension. This negatively reinforces smoking as a means of reducing anxiety. Physiologically, nicotine is a stimulant, which actually raises anxiety.

I once worked with a woman who loved to sing and had a great laugh but who bit off pieces of her own fingers when her anxiety and subsequent frustration peaked. When she shook your hand, she was missing parts of three fingers.

Most cutting is non-suicidal. When tension and stress builds up, it gets released at the moment of self-injurious behavior. The pain provides a temporary release from this anxiety build-up that is "worth it." One of my clients used a hot iron or the ends of an electrical cord to pick or cut her skin. I worked with one man who ate glass or tire when he got anxious. Yes, these are extreme examples, but they demonstrate the power of negative reinforcement. Like relief from a headache, people are after "Relief" from the emotional pain.

FACILITATING SOME FORMS THAT ARE HEALING

Some forms of negative reinforcement–anxiety reduction via avoidance–are helpful in alleviating unnecessary problems. Many veterans avoid VA medical centers for a range of reasons including treatment angst, the mental health stigma, or anxiety about "having to talk about what happened." In recent years, a VA in the Midwest had landscaping issues, because the greenery resembled areas of Vietnam. In this case, it would have been better to have veterans come into the hospital and do exposures in controlled therapeutic settings than have some untreated Vietnam vets suffer and drive away. In another example, the principal of the school at Columbine spent many hours after the massacre changing the sounds of the emergency alarm in order to avoid eliciting intense fear and panic.

ANXIETY REDUCERS CAN NEGATIVELY REINFORCE ANXIETY

Xanax reduces anxiety in the short-term, but reinforces anxiety in the long-term. It is not uncommon for people to convince themselves that sensations like chest pressure, heart palpitations, and trembling require Xanax. This belief also gets reinforced when a person rushes to the hospital believing, "I am having a heart attack." Heart or thyroid problems can resemble panic symptoms and these need to be assessed with regular physical exams.

Repeat visits to get blood tests to check thyroids and other possible conditions are often anxiety-related. Likewise, heart tests such as electrocardiograms (ECG or EKG) result from panic attacks leading to ER visits. It is common for clients with panic symptoms to make multiple ER visits. One woman stated that she was told by an ER not to return because "I was told I have anxiety" after she went to the ER believing she had heart problems on five occasions during a three-month period.

NRBs AS HEAVY-, MIDDLE-, OR LIGHTWEIGHTS

In the assessment of negative reinforcement behaviors (NRB's), therapists can view their severity as heavyweights, middleweights, and lightweights based how much they reinforce and sustain anxiety. Xanax and ER visits are two of the heavyweights of negative reinforcement. A 6-ounce flask that would have four 1.5-ounce shots of vodka is another strong form but a middleweight, unless alcoholism is a prominent comorbid disorder. Other middleweights include taking a "safe person" to an outing. Other examples of middleweight negative reinforcement include rushing straight to the shoe aisle with set criteria ("these three things, then I'm out of here") or leaving the store prematurely when panic symptoms develop for someone with agoraphobia. Checking one's pulse, Facebook page and checking emails or tweets are all anxiety reducers that can actually reinforce anxiety. Essentially, anything that serves as a distraction and avoidance tactic and influences a person to avoid taking things head-on have a negative reinforcement effect. The goal is exposure–not avoidance.

Prayer can be a form of anxiety reducer that reinforces anxiety if it coincides with avoidance. I once worked with a college freshman named Houa who had social anxiety. As we talked, it became evident that she would avoid meetings and pray as she did so. During one incident, right before she went into an Asian Association meeting, she turned around and walked away. As she turned around, she began praying the Lord's Prayer. Intervention included a cognitive reframing which involved seeing prayer as associated with empowering her to face her challenges rather than to reinforce her avoidance of them.

Examples of lightweight NRB's include cracking knuckles, nail-biting, saying "ums" or "uhs," or jerking while walking through a doorway (a man was unable to identify the origin of this behavior but did it as a way of safety seeking; he felt anxious when he didn't jerk).

Safety-seeking behaviors negatively reinforce anxiety. Research shows that safety-seeking behaviors cause anxiety to persist (Dunmore, Clark, & Ehlers, 2001; Sloan & Telch, 2002). They bring temporary relief but sustain beliefs that drive anxiety. A person who relies on the use of maps in a grocery store reinforces the belief that she is incompetent without a path to follow in and out of the aisles. Likewise, alcohol is often used as a security blanket when visiting with family members during the holidays. The long-term goal in anxiety treatment is to help clients eliminate safety-seeking behavior and forms of negative reinforcement.

Severity	Examples of Negative Reinforcement Behaviors (NRBs)
Heavyweights	Xanax and ER Visits
Middleweights	Taking a "safety person," avoidance behaviors, checking, superstitious behavior, reassurance seeking, holding onto objects
Lightweights	Distraction rituals, nail biting

ASSESSMENT VERSUS INTERVENTION

Good evaluations include assessing for negative reinforcement in the life of your client or patient. This involves identifying behaviors that negatively reinforce anxiety. These are all avoidant types of behavior as well as safety behaviors.

Jill with healthy anxiety may spend many hours searching the internet for information that would confirm that a particular skin rash is benign and not a sign of melanoma. By assessing for this type of NRB, a therapist can help Jill reduce her internet searches which only serve to strengthen her catastrophic beliefs (i.e. worst case health scenario).

Shannon with panic disorder only traveled to the store with a close family member. By engaging in this NRB, she fails to learn that she will not have a heart attack from the chest pressure she feels when she gets anxious. Thus, because of her reliance on her NRB, her catastrophic fear belief is not disconfirmed. After identifying the safety behavior, the first step in the assessment process is – what would happen if you didn't bring the "safety person" to the store? What could you do to tolerate the anxiety?

The intervention component of NRBs involves collaborating with the client on reducing safety-seeking behaviors: reassurance seeking, checking, having immediate access to medications, holding onto objects, being with a safety person, and other aforementioned examples.

ACTIONS THAT REFRAME EXAGGERATIONS

The third part of becoming unafraid is reframing exaggerated threat appraisals. Practicing reappraisals is the most direct approach and often involves bringing balanced thinking into a client's tendency to magnify problems. In this chapter, behavioral experiments do something that has the same effect as a depressive that gets up, lets the light in and goes for a walk. Actions can speak change louder than words.

Reframing exaggerated threat appraisals often requires actions to reduce anxiety. Consider the following anxiety-producing beliefs: "I can't stand the anxiety;" "When my heart starts to beat faster, I dread the feeling;" "I can't stand to take risks; it's better to be safe than sorry;" "I detest shopping for groceries,

> *I believe half the unhappiness in life comes from people being afraid to go straight at things.*
>
> William J. Lock

especially when my sister is not able to go with me;" "I hate that nausea feeling in the pit of my stomach that triggers further panic feelings."

Sometimes it is helpful for therapists to encourage clients toward self-direction actions that help them gather evidence through experience that disconfirms their belief. Another aspect of anxiety tolerance is encouraging clients to do experiments that help them reframe their anxiety-producing beliefs. The experiments require a level of anxiety tolerance that the client will need to be prepared for. As mentioned, exposure is about readiness. When doing experiments to gather evidence, anxiety goes up.

Phase one involves identifying those anxiety producing thoughts that elicit the highest levels of anxiety on scales (0-10 or SUDS: 0-100). Phase two involves taking experimental actions that challenge those beliefs.

> *Change is not made without inconvenience, even from worse to better.*
>
> Richard Hooker

Anxiety-Producing Belief	Experimental Action
"It would be horrible if I were to look anxious in a social situation."	Pour water all over your head, practice shaking your hands, practice having breathing difficulties, appear anxious while in a public area. Do people seem to notice?
"If someone sees my home when it's dirty, they will call me a lazy slob."	Make your house a complete mess, and invite your neighbors or friends. Did anyone indicate negativity?
"My house will burn down if I don't check the stove 14 times an evening."	Don't check your stove at all for one day and see if you're alive in the morning.
"If I ask others for help, they will think I'm an idiot."	Ask another adult if they will show you how to pump gas. Did anyone call you an idiot?

Phase 3 involves the therapist and client processing about the effectiveness of the action taken. Was there any discomfort? What was your anxiety level on a scale of 0-10? If avoidance occurred, addressing the degree to which the belief was strengthened. "That is O.K., you may not have been ready yet. The key is readiness." Once avoidance is extinguished and action is taken, therapists provide praise for courageous exposure and continue to help clients reframe their exaggerated beliefs.

CHAPTER 5

Changing the World One Thought at a Time: Reclaiming Core Beliefs

PSYCHOTHERAPY RESEARCH IS GOLDEN

For a brief moment, let's take a look at the last 60 years of psychotherapy research. This summary is obviously a condensed version of the journey taken in the field of study on psychological treatment.

While Landis (1937) and Denker (1946) raised questions regarding the effectiveness of psychotherapy, it was British psychologist Hans Eysenck (1952) who said that the psychotherapies in widest use at the time were largely ineffective and useless. Studies "fail to prove that psychotherapy, Freudian or otherwise, facilitates the recovery of neurotic patients" (1952, p. 323). In response to harsh critiques of the methodology in the studies he evaluated, Eysenck (1960) came to the same conclusions with better-designed and more reliably controlled studies. This critique propelled therapists to demonstrate with empirical evidence that what they do is beneficial.

Over the years, several studies emerged as attempts to prove that psychotherapy is beneficial. A notably significant paper by Luborsky, Singer, and Luborsky (1976) compared an assortment of outcomes from a variety of treatments: group versus individual

> There are two kinds of truth: the truth that lights the way and the truth that warms the heart. The first of these is science, and the second is art. Neither is independent of the other or more important than the other. Without art science would be as useless as a pair of high forceps in the hands of a plumber. Without science art would become a crude mess of folklore and emotional quackery. The truth of art keeps science from becoming inhuman, and the truth of science keeps art from becoming ridiculous.
>
> Raymond Chandler

psychotherapy, time-limited versus open-ended psychotherapy, and client-centered versus traditional psychotherapy approaches. This study concluded that all forms of psychotherapy are beneficial.

But, more empirical evidence remained a necessity. A year later, Smith and Glass (1977) established a new statistical procedure, called the meta-analysis, in order to determine the effectiveness of psychotherapy. The meta-analysis is a method of synthesizing the results of independent studies. In 1977, Smith and Glass's meta-analyses of large numbers of outcome studies showed treatment increasing psychological health and healing. As the years passed, many academicians collaborated with practitioners to establish improved psychotherapy research.

The 1995 APA division 12 list of empirically validated treatments was an important work in the field (Task Force, 1995). While some people argue this was a way to justify psychological treatments for managed care companies who were looking to cut mental health care, the list established efficacy treatments for practitioners.

Several researchers attempted to engage in the discussion of what was needed in research including Foa and Meadows (1997) who articulated the seven "gold standards" for research design including clearly defined symptoms and reliable and valid measures. As time passed, criteria that were established for empirically supported treatments included at least two good between-group design experiments that demonstrated efficacy using treatment manuals, specified characteristics of client samples, and effects demonstrated by at least two different investigators (or investigation teams).

EMPIRICAL GUIDANCE COMES FROM TREATMENT GUIDES & META-ANALYSES

In recent years, guides and books have emerged with established lists of treatments based on gold standard psychotherapy research (Nathan & Gorman, 2007; Roth & Fonagy, 2005), particularly for anxiety treatment (DeRubeis, Brotman, & Gibbons, 2005). Research on psychological interventions continues to explode with 150 meta-analyses published between 2011 and 2013, including a meta-analysis of imagery rehearsal and CBT for insomnia resulting in greater improvement in sleep quality (Casement & Swanson, 2012); or results showing empathy as a moderately strong predictor of therapy outcome for 59 independent samples and 3,599 clients (Elliott, Bohart, Watson, & Greenberg, 2011); or a meta-analysis showing cognitive therapy (CT) for pathological worry in adults with GAD resulted in 57%

of participants classed as recovered at 12 months following CT completion (Hanrahan, Field, Jones, & Davey, 2013).

The most relevant meta-analyses that form the bedrock for this book have been those studies that identify successful treatment for anxiety. Meta-analyses have indicated that cognitive and behavioral techniques reduce symptoms of panic disorder (Gould, Otto, & Pollack, 1995; Mitte, 2005), generalized anxiety disorder (Gould, Otto, Pollack, & Yap, 1997), social phobia (Taylor, 1996), obsessive–compulsive disorder (Abramowitz, 1997) and posttraumatic stress disorder (Foa, Hembree, & Cahill, 2005).

COMMON VERSUS SPECIFIC FACTORS

For decades, the debate was about theoretical orientation. The questions that emerged from these research discussions transitioned to what treatments work for what types of individuals and what types of problems and disorders. Variables analyzed in therapy include matching therapist characteristics, treatment, and patient characteristics (Beutler, & Harwood, 2000). The APA Evidence Based Practice Task Force (2005), using the established definition of empirically-based practice developed by the Institute of Medicine (2001),

> *It's a bit embarrassing to have been concerned with the human problem all one's life and find at the end that one has no more to offer by way of advice than 'Try to be a little kinder.'*
>
> Aldous Huxley

emphasized these variables when reviewing the research evidence: psychological interventions, clinical expertise, and an assessment of the patient's characteristics, preferences, and context. Many factors have been considered as determinants of therapy effectiveness. Some argue that client factors are the most influential determinant in therapy outcome (Orlinsky, Ronnestand, & Willutzki, 2004; Duncan, Miller, Wampold, & Hubble, 2010). Basically, if a client is motivated to get better, therapy outcome exponentially improves.

In clinical research, the essential debate in its simplified form over the last 15 years has transitioned to common versus specific factors. Common factors are those factors common to all treatments: empathic listening, unconditional positive regard, compassion, and the strength of the therapeutic relationship. Specific factors are those factors specific to the types of treatment: cognitive restructuring, exposure and response prevention, interoceptive exposure, and social skills training. Essentially, what is more important–the relationship or the treatment method? Every group of practitioners that I speak to in my seminars answer "both."

NECESSARY BUT NOT SUFFICIENT

Carl Rogers said the therapeutic relationship is necessary and sufficient (1957). The unforgettable Aaron Beck took a different position. He said the relationship is necessary but not sufficient (1979). As an aside, Albert Ellis stated that the therapeutic relationship is neither necessary, nor sufficient (1962). On a humorous note, I went to Albert Ellis's memorial service several years ago and Beck stated to the large audience that Ellis actually liked his patients. The audience laughed in unison because Ellis was notorious for a harsh and confrontational therapeutic style.

The idea that the therapeutic relationship is necessary but not sufficient is rooted in the idea that psychological treatment is more than just chit-chat (i.e. advice talk with wise Aunt Ruth). And, it is more than providing warmth, establishing relationship rapport, and providing a knowledge base of psychological expertise (i.e. a well read and kind academician).

ASSUMING THE RELATIONSHIP...

I learned a valuable relationship lesson in college from my advisor Dr. John Buri, a relationship expert and authority on learning and memory: "Assume nothing and communicate everything." So, for the following to be true, plenty of communication would have been needed in the therapeutic relationship for the following assumptions.

> For two personalities to meet is like mixing two chemical substances. If there is any combination at all, both are transformed.
>
> Carl Jung

Let's assume the therapist recognizes and values the importance of the therapeutic relationship, which is critical for successful therapy (Fluckiger, Del Re, Wampold, Symonds, & Horvath, 2012). Let's assume you process in the therapy; this involves noticing relational behaviors in therapy, and inquiring if the client does this in their relationships outside of therapy. For example, if Carrie changes the subject in session when she is uncomfortable, inquiring from Carrie how this behavior pattern occurs in other relationships can help raise insight about her behavioral patterns. When a client shuts down or withdraws emotionally, discussing this behavior in therapy and connecting to similar behavior outside of therapy is part of the therapy process. If a client struggles with being vulnerable in therapy, then this challenge may be evident with important relationships as well. Discussing these pertinent behaviors may be relevant to the treatment plan. This may also involve addressing defensiveness and the client's use of defensive maneuvers. The notion of "therapist adjustment" is a skill that refers to how a therapist adjusts interventions in accordance with the client's defensive maneuvers (Despland, de Roten, Despars, Stigler, and Perry, 2001).

Let's assume the therapist expresses good counseling micro-skills: empathic listening, words of encouragement, helpful paraphrasing, accurate summarizations, open and closed questions with good timing, warmth, unconditional positive regard, and compassion. Good therapy involves helping patients cultivate more compassion toward themselves to reduce and replace self-criticalness (Gilbert & Irons, 2005; Schanche, 2013).

Let's assume the therapist communicates with hope and optimism and empathically responds to the client's emotional pain. Many clients have few people (or nobody) who believes in them. One of the best gifts a therapist can give their clients is belief in who they are and what they can do. This may involve belief in change or belief that the person can overcome current trials and tribulations. This can involve instilling hope, which is a substantial strength builder, or encouragement emphasizing that past memories are not today's realities. A good therapist also incorporates client preferences in a collaborative goal-setting process. Therapists can improve client satisfaction when presenting a treatment rationale by addressing clients' outcome expectations (Swift & Derthick, 2013), which explain 15% of the variance in treatment outcomes (Norcross & Lambert, 2011).

THE SOCRATIC TREATMENT METHOD

If the therapeutic relationship with deeply felt compassion is necessary, what else in therapy is necessary and sufficient for an effective outcome? In the treatment of anxiety disorders, it is the treatment method. This chapter tackles the most essential elements of the cognitive therapy treatment method.

Socratic questioning involves identifying the evidence behind the thoughts. What evidence supports this thought? On the other side of things, what evidence is against it being true? What could be another explanation or interpretation of the situation? Why else did it happen? What is the best and worst outcome in this situation? What is the

> *You can tell whether people are clever by their answers. You can tell whether people are wise by their questions.*
>
> Naguib Mahfouz, 1988
> Nobel Prize for Literature

most bearable outcome? In terms of tolerance, could you tolerate the worst-case scenario? These are the types of traditional sets of questions that help bring clearness to muddled problems. Then there are decisions–what are the advantages and disadvantages of taking the risk? Is not acting is a calculated decision based on risk assessment?

DRAWING OUT CORE BELIEFS FOR THERAPY

There are several questions that help draw out core beliefs for therapy. During the experience, what was going through your mind? Or (future) what's likely going to go through your mind? What is the most central belief about yourself? What went through your mind when you didn't get the job? What

> *Every sentence that I utter should be regarded by you not as an assertion but as a question.*
>
> Niels Bohr, Nobel Prize in Physics

words help you express your negative belief about yourself now?

There are four central negative belief (NB) categories that most anxiety problems arise from: (1) defective – effective category, (2) degree of responsibility category, (3) control – freedom category, and (4) the trust – safety category. Five crucial strategies to disarm and transform these four central negative belief categories are identified in this book: open chair technique, safe place guided imagery, role playing technique, a time machine technique, and straight forward evidence-gathering using Socratic questioning.

IDENTIFYING THE FIRST OF FOUR CENTRAL NB AREAS

The first of four central negative belief (NB) categories that most anxiety problems arise from consists of (1) how people think about who they are at the core. This consists of their internal dialogue, self-talk, and self-whisperings. This inner thought life manifests in self-esteem and self-efficacy. At the very core, what are your beliefs about you? How a person sees himself or herself results from the family of origin and early childhood experiences in addition to all nurturing experiences along the way. This category (1) is described as defective-effective and targets key cognitions such as self-worth, one's view of how lovable one is, and how much one deserves love. This category is unrelated to socioeconomic status, professional status, or educational background. It is unrelated to external circumstances or material privileges. It is entirely related to how clients see themselves—as a bad person or

> *The greatest challenge to any thinker is stating the problem in a way that will allow a solution.*
>
> Bertrand Russell

a loving person, insignificant or a person of significance. The high-powered executive and the homeless addict both have their individualized hang-ups (NBs); the former probably found ways to compensate with achievements and education more effectively.

> *Don't let someone else's opinion of you become your reality.*
>
> Les Brown

I Am Defective – I Am Effective Category

Negative Belief (NB)	Reframed Belief (RB)
I am worthless.	I am worthy.
I am unlovable.	I am lovable.
I don't deserve love.	I deserve love.
I am stupid.	I am intelligent.
I am insignificant.	I am significant.
I deserve to be miserable.	I deserve to be happy.
I am a bad person.	I am a loving person.
I deserve to die.	I deserve to live.

Not Limited To Lonely, Uneducated...

These beliefs are not limited to the lonely, uneducated, unemployed, homeless, or individuals in despair. For many, these defective beliefs underlie their overcompensating behavior. Surprisingly, this is seen in very accomplished individuals: PhDs, MDs, attorneys, bankers, politicians, and professors. How many of us become psychologists, professional counselors, or social workers to compensate for our own thoughts of inadequacy? You know the type–"I heard 'you'll never amount to anything,' and I set out to prove him wrong." Examples of compensating occur in a variety of ways. Consider the expert statistician who was made fun of for his math as a kid. Or, a prominent vegan nutritionist whose father managed processed foods in a vending machine business. Or the politician whose dad laughed at his stuttering. On the surface, these are examples of individuals who overcame their challenges. For some, their defective beliefs are buried under their successful exteriors.

I worked with a woman named Jacqueline, a pre-med college student. She had two older brothers who were physicians. Both of her parents were physicians. Her grandparents were physicians. When I saw her, she presented with a problem of test anxiety, and it became clear quickly that her test performance was not due to lack of knowledge in the particular tested areas. Her perfectionism was causing problems for her test results. She had unrelenting standards and was hypercritical. Jacqueline thought it was unacceptable to make a mistake, which only elevated her anxiety. She experienced great pressure and worried constantly about the ramifications of "not making it" influenced by her family background. Her core belief wasn't "I am stupid." She knew she was good enough to make it, and her intellectual capacity was not going to limit her. Over time during the course of therapy, her primary negative belief that emerged was "I am unlovable." She pointed out behavior patterns in her family where she was loved conditionally depending upon her achievements. In a high achievement family such as Jacqueline's, it is common for an individual's self-worth to be primarily based on achievement, rather than who they are. This was true in Jacqueline's case–her feeling of self-worth was based on achievement.

> *We've been all the way to the moon and back, but have trouble crossing the street to meet a new neighbor. We conquered outer space but not inner space. We've done larger things, but no better things.*
>
> George Carlin

> *We have multiplied our possessions, but reduced our values. We talk too much, love too seldom, and hate too often. We've learned how to make a living, but not a life; we've added years to life, not life to years.*
>
> George Carlin

USING THE OPEN CHAIR TECHNIQUE TO REFRAME

I've talked with two young adults in pre-med who both went in opposite directions based on their own personal experience outside of therapy. One young man (let's call him Joe) was in the mountains of Colorado on the other side of Pikes Peak when he experienced what he called an epiphany. The idea became clear to him that he was "being called" to be a doctor and he decided to pursue pre-med, enter medical school, and (many years later) became a doctor. In contrast, a college student named Ann was already a pre-med student and went on a "global semester" where she took classes and traveled to 15 different countries. When she saw children in India, she was so moved by the experience that she decided to forgo medical school and travel and teach children in other countries. She went on to teach in China.

In both examples, these two individuals described the experiences as epiphanies that changed their lives. While somewhat orchestrated, the experiential strategy of the open chair technique can have a similar type of emotional impact if done at the appropriate time. I used it with Jacqueline to elicit emotional experience and help obtain clarity in her mind as to what she wanted from her family and how she views herself now. In session, another chair was positioned with the appropriate space from Jacqueline. Before we began, she was invited to identify the person she most wanted to talk to about love being conditional and based on achievement.

In her case, she said it was her father who came across as "inflexible." She thought he only got excited "when I won something or accomplished something." Jacqueline went on to share with her father as the tears flowed.

> Too many of us are not living our dreams because we are living our fears.
>
> Les Brown

I allowed Jacqueline to lead the way. The only cue that was given was inviting her to share with the chair (and her visualized father) what she wanted him to believe about her. This was a powerful experience when Jacqueline shared with her father that she wanted him to see her as lovable. After the session, she was asked "what was that like?" In subsequent sessions, we discussed the experience. One of the key breakthroughs for Jacqueline was when she scaled her belief from 0 -10, from "I am unlovable" to "I am lovable" in terms of what she believes about herself now. She scaled a 10 and communicated that her rationale was that "she doesn't need confirmation from others for her own confidence and identity."

Oh yeah, her presenting problem. As therapy came to a close, her test anxiety decreased significantly. She also reported less pressure to perform, more enjoyment and satisfaction with her studies, and more of a 'personal calling' rather than an 'external controlled calling.'

IDENTIFYING THE SECOND OF FOUR CENTRAL NB AREAS

The second central negative belief (NB) category from which anxiety problems arise is related to the degree of responsibility. When it comes to a person's relationship with time, these NBs are related to things that

> I never learn anything talking. I only learn things when I ask questions.
>
> Lou Holtz

have happened in the past—to decisions made and to behavior patterns like parenting, and relationships. These are most commonly regrets. A common regret I hear from lonely geriatric patients is wishing they had children.

If you notice the negative beliefs in this category, they are consistent with "shoulds" and how life "should" have gone or how I "should" have chosen the right path. Upon reflection, it is more advantageous and empowering to modify the shoulds to preferences. Thus, I would have preferred to have known better, but I learned from my mistakes. I would have preferred to have been a better parent but I did the best I could. The reframing of negative beliefs in the degree of responsibility category consists of two phases: (1) changing the shoulds to preferences and (2) the reality-based empowering reframe. The reframed beliefs below are examples, but there are infinite possibilities that need to be individualized for each client.

DEGREE OF RESPONSIBILITY CATEGORY

Negative Belief (NB)	Reframed Belief (RB)
I should have known better.	I learned from my mistakes.
I should have been a better parent.	I did the best I could.
I should have left the relationship earlier.	I can learn from my decisions to be a better decision maker.
I should have stayed committed to the relationship.	I can learn from my decisions.

USING THE ROLE-PLAYING TECHNIQUE ON "SHOULDS"

In this intervention, the client is invited to think about a friend or a trusted confidant while the central "should" belief is identified. The client identifies the person from the past or present whom they trust the most. The choice of the trusted confidant is explored with questions like the following: In what way have they earned your trust? In what ways are you grateful to them?

The client is then invited to put themselves in their trusted confidant's shoes (traditionally referred to as "distancing"). While considering the negative "should belief;" What advice would the confidant give? There are many situations in which advice from trusted others is helpful if heeded. The purpose of this role-playing is to think differently. I like to use another chair in this process.

IDENTIFYING THE THIRD OF FOUR CENTRAL NB AREAS

The third central negative belief (NB) category from which anxiety problems arise is the control versus freedom category. These beliefs are primarily relationally based. When a couple comes into my office, the degree of relational health is often dependent on the degree of freedom within the partnership. Is each person free to express their emotions? Is each partner free to talk about sources of stress? Openness of communication is related to the degree of control within the relationship.

Freedom from fear is what this book is all about. Many clients controlled by fear have been controlled by others. Beliefs such as powerlessness, inadequacy, helplessness, failure, and imperfection are all related to being heavily controlled in past relationships by parents, partners, and even teachers and bosses. Professional work environments with micro-managers can have a powerful effect on somebody's interpretation of their freedom, particularly if they don't perceive themselves as having other job options. "I am not in control" and "he controls me" are negative beliefs that squelch freedom and conditions people to remain trapped in feared emotional states.

CONTROL VERSUS FREEDOM CATEGORY

Negative Belief (NB)	Reframed Belief (RB)
I am not in control.	I am now in control of my life.
I am powerless.	I am powerful and I have choices.
I am a failure.	I can succeed.
I have to be perfect.	I can be myself and accept my mistakes.
My life is dictated and cannot be changed.	I am free to change my life.
I am inadequate.	I am capable and strong.
He / She controls me.	I have immense freedom.
I am helpless.	I have personal power to help my situation.

"I AM NOT IN CONTROL"

I worked with a businessman named Sal who came into therapy for "extraordinary stress." He was working 80 hours per week and was referred by a colleague to "get a little more balanced." My initial impression was that Sal was looking for some quick tips so he could jam even more work in with less sleep. His face showed a disappointed reaction when I suggested getting more sleep. Sal was obsessed with work and appeared as an overachiever by ceaselessly driving himself. Unfortunately, he showed only poor to fair insight into his problems and showed little realization of the cost of his excessive work and its consequences on his family. He would be sitting at his kid's soccer game and check and send work email the entire time, according to his wife's complaint.

> *The best years of your life are the ones in which you decide your problems are your own. You do not blame them on your mother, the ecology, or the president. You realize that you control your own destiny.*
>
> Albert Ellis

One of the cognitions that emerged during the course of therapy was: "I am not in control." His interpretation of his work was that it was out of his control and he felt like prey to his budget, his boss, his fears about the future and the economy, and his anxiety about competition in the workplace.

UNPACKING THE DEEPER CORE BELIEF

During the course of Sal's therapy, key issues discussed included getting balanced, incorporating exercise, improving sleep hygiene, attending to his fatherhood. Stress management strategies included problem-solving under stress through the use of deep breathing exercises. The deeper core belief that was unpacked was identifying his failure schema. He revealed that his father informed him that he would be a failure in life. Sal looked like he was punched in the gut when I asked him how this related to his excessive work habits.

USING SAFE PLACE GUIDED IMAGERY

I asked Sal to close his eyes and picture himself in a safe place. I invited him to just let an image of a safe place come into his mind. Here are some of the questions that followed: What do you see? What sounds do you hear? Does it have a smell? What about that picture allows you to feel peace as the stress leaves your body? Can you describe the colors that you see in your mind? In addition to the questions, Sal was taught to notice using mindfulness. Notice the sounds that you hear. Notice the colors that you see. Notice the feelings in your body. Notice your breath. Notice the beauty of the safe place.

In the second series of imagery exercises, Sal was asked to see himself as a boy in the safe place. He was then invited to see his father in the safe place.

What would you have wanted your father to say to you then that he didn't say to you? Among a number of things, Sal stated that he would have wanted his father to tell him that he would be a success with whatever he put his hands on to do.

> Life is not measured by the number of breaths we take, but by the moments that take our breath away.
>
> George Carlin

He decided that he didn't need to spend his life proving his father wrong and compensating for his failure schema. When I saw him for a follow-up session, he stated that his wife was happier although she still thought he worked too much (down to 60 hours). He did state that he was off on weekends and never touched his Blackberry at his son's soccer games.

IDENTIFYING THE FOURTH CENTRAL NB AREA

It is common for clients who have experienced abuse to have difficulty trusting others. If a child touches the hot burner and gets hurt, arms will stay recoiled for a long time. Trusting others is similar. It is common to cope in one of three unhealthy ways following hurts: (1) repeatedly enter into hurtful relationships, (2) avoid relationships altogether, or (3) become bitter and abuse or hurt others.

Those who enter into hurtful relationships are those clients who cope by surrendering to their personal experience. Their emotional learning and hijacking influence these types of individuals. In many cases, this entails an emotional crippling by small or big Ts. Boys who have

> At no time in history has so large a proportion of humanity rated love so highly.
>
> Morton M. Hunt

been physically harmed by their dads commonly become bitter and hurt others. It is common for these boys to do similar things to physically assert dominance when they become fathers to their sons (and girls when they become mothers, too). More than surrendering to hurtful relationships or becoming hurtful, the most common strategy for those who have been hurt is to avoid. Avoidance is the primary strategy due to mistrust and "feeling unsafe."

The more healthy strategies following hurts and emotional experiences that breed mistrust is coming to a recognition of one's ability to trust again. Or, learning to be more selective in whom to trust. This is also connected to interior self-talk and beliefs about trusting themselves.

TRUST – MISTRUST AND SAFE – UNSAFE CATEGORY

Negative Belief (NB)	Reframed Belief (RB)
I cannot be assertive.	I can learn to make my needs known.
I am in danger.	It's over. I am safe now. It is not happening right now.
I will abuse others' trust.	I have the ability to maintain the trust of others.
I cannot trust anyone.	I can choose whom to trust.
I cannot be trusted.	I can be trusted. I am capable of responsible decision-making.
I cannot trust my judgment.	I can trust my judgment.
I cannot be independent; I cannot be safe on my own.	I can learn to take care of myself.

TAKING RISKS WITH YOUR MISTRUST

Yoda said "you must unlearn what you have learned." Yoda's advice on unlearning is most difficult in the area of emotional vulnerability. One of the most difficult areas of vulnerability is in the area of trust. Individuals who have

> *In time we hate that which we often fear.*
>
> William Shakespeare

been divorced talk about the enormous energy required to try to date again. Twenty-year faithful employees cut during the latest economic recession talk about the daunting effort to find replacement work with their ruptured trust. Clients with clinical issues have trouble going to a "therapist" and talking to a "stranger" because of anxiety due to mistrust.

I recently saw a 50-year old woman (Beth) who is coping with fibromyalgia, post-polio syndrome with right side pain in her leg, foot, and ankle, migraine headaches, and chronic fatigue. She experienced her first panic attack three years ago and thought she "was having a heart attack and rushed to the hospital." As an aside, when I ask therapists at seminars if they work with a client who has rushed to the hospital frightened of having a heart attack, nearly everyone raises their hand. When Beth first started out in therapy, she stated: "I hate people." In addition to continued medical care, she required treatment for her panic disorder. When she began to settle down

> *If the highest aim of a captain were to preserve his ship, he would keep it in port forever.*
>
> Thomas Aquinas

in a supportive and empathic therapeutic relationship, the meaning of the "hate" that she expressed was less obscured, and it became clear she was really expressing mistrust.

MAKING USE OF THE TIME MACHINE TECHNIQUE

This technique is a simple way of preparing for the future. I call it resource installation for the future. Someone like Beth tells herself in advance what people will be like and then confirms those beliefs in her own mind when she meets them. This issue is addressed with the time machine technique. To jump ahead in time, Beth is encouraged to visualize a highly distressing possibility in the future (near or distant future). In session, Beth is invited to expound on details of a hypothetical scenario. As an aside, the scenario has to be representative of a likely stressor, not something so outlandish and unlikely. While visualizing this scenario, Beth is asked what would need to happen for her to begin to believe that she can choose whom to trust. When Beth was resistant, I said "I am not saying that you will believe this. But, if you were to believe it, what evidence do you have in your life right now that this is a possibility."

SUCCESS IN SMALL STEPS

Beth began to take small steps to spend time with others. During the course of therapy, she began to realize that she was angry at herself for "wrong" relationship choices. She believed that she couldn't trust her own judgment based on these decisions. However, as time passed, her small steps of success led to her beginning to see that she could make responsible decisions, trust her own judgment, and begin to be selective about who she spent time with. In terms of her treatment plan, she stopped withdrawing, increased her assertiveness, was less angry at herself and others, more tolerant of her panic feelings which lessened their frequency and impact, and was compliant with her medical treatment believing others were actually interested in helping her.

ONE OF THE BEST LONG-TERM GIFTS IS META-COGNITION AND THE REFLECTIVE LIFE

As a final thought for this chapter, my friend once told me: "you can't lead a person to a place you aren't willing to go yourself." The context of this comment was self-reflection on core issues in one's interior life. In other words, therapists try to help clients eliminate self-deception and to be honest with themselves. To do this well, as therapists we need to continuously peel back our onions as well. And, discussing the value of meta-cognition and the reflective life is a great gift.

In my experience, there are three key elements to engaging in reflectiveness: time set aside, good reading, and good friends. One key element of a reflective life is to actually set aside time–with the busy-ness of life, few people actually take the time to reflect. The second key to reflectiveness is reading. What is read can trigger reflection, insights, and understanding. Also, good movies can increase reflectiveness. Third, good friends who help us think about life help increase meta-cognition and the reflective life.

CHAPTER 6

Developing a Freedom Lifestyle with Optimal Health

A Healthy Lifestyle Diminishes the Power of Anxiety

There are three things that I often point to when I talk with clients working to overcome their anxiety: good sleep hygiene, healthy eating habits, and regular exercise. These areas are goals for everybody seeking to live a healthy and optimally balanced lifestyle. And, it is these three areas that often take a back seat in the busy-ness of life.

> *I've always believed that if you put in the work, the results will come.*
>
> Michael Jordan

Overcoming Insomnia

One of the effects of anxiety disorders is insomnia. A man I saw who survived being shot in a drive-by had difficulty staying asleep because of distressing dreams. A college student with a pre-med major had difficulty falling asleep because of her self-doubt and racing thoughts. Some people experience difficulty falling asleep due to anxiety. Others tend to wake prematurely or wake up multiple times throughout the night.

I have used sleep diaries with a variety of patients from PTSD survivors and addicts to college students. When individuals take the time to reflect on their own sleep, they often gain valuable awareness. Below is a sample of how you can record some baseline information about your sleep patterns. Enter the information before bed and when you get up, total hours of sleep, and any medications taken. Adjust from time to bed to time to sleep and time you woke from time you stepped out of bed.

SLEEP DIARY				
Date	Time to Sleep	Time of Awakening	Total Sleep	Medication Used

SLEEP MEDICATION IS PROBLEMATIC LONG-TERM

Sleep problems are a result of disrupted circadian rhythms. For a person with anxiety, increased arousal and worry prevents sleep. After a while, this wakefulness alters circadian rhythms. Sleeping pills like Ativan or Trazadone alter your circadian rhythms in a non-natural way. Sleeping pills help with sleep in the short-term but they don't reverse insomnia naturally to obtain a stable state of equilibrium. Research shows that cognitive behavioral therapy (i.e. behavioral sleep medicine) is far more effective than sleeping pills for improving sleep and reversing insomnia long-term. Before you make any changes in medication, talk with your physician.

REVERSING INSOMNIA

1. Achieve *a consistent sleep cycle*. This involves going to bed and getting up at the same time. Now, expecting college students to go to bed at 10:00 p.m. and getting up at 6:00 a.m. is unrealistic. But, some modification of a 4 a.m. bedtime may be doable. The goal is to develop a regular sleep time.

> It is health that is real wealth and not pieces of gold and silver.
>
> Mahatma Gandhi

2. Take the *television out of the bedroom*. The majority of people, including children, have TVs in their bedroom. When I am speaking, I always ask for a show of hands of those who have TVs in their bedrooms, and I always get the majority of the audience. When people use the bed for watching television, reading, texting, tweeting, using Snapchat® or Facebook®, they are associating the bed with arousal and anxiety. It is best for the bed to be used for only sleep (and sex). Nothing else!

3. *Eliminate Naps.* Naps disrupt your circadian rhythms. When people nap, they are more likely to fall asleep later or increase awakenings. This is difficult for many people because naps make you feel good. The goal is to obtain consistency with bedtime and wake-up time. Also, the more consistent the sleep schedule, the more likely you will get up naturally in the morning without the need for an alarm.

4. *Reduce Consumption.* Sleep is often disturbed by need for the bathroom. Avoid caffeine products, fats, sugar (that is you, ice cream lovers!), and alcohol. I

> The first wealth is health.
>
> Ralph Waldo Emerson

talk to a lot of people who use alcohol as a sleep aid and they believe it makes them sleep better. As a depressant, it may assist with falling asleep. But, it becomes an integrated stimulant after several hours and produces awakenings.

5. *Practice Progressive Relaxation.* Progressive relaxation is a behavioral intervention that reduces tension and increases relaxation. It involves tightening up muscle groups and then releasing them while noticing the difference between tension and relaxation. Here is a sample sequence of muscle groups that can be followed. Take some deep breathes from

> A vigorous five-mile walk will do more good for an unhappy but otherwise healthy adult than all the medicine and psychology in the world.
>
> Paul Dudley White

the core abdomen. As you breathe deeply, make sure the stomach goes out when you inhale (not the chest or shoulders). True diaphragmatic breathing involves inhaling and exhaling from the core. Then hold a muscle group for 15 seconds before releasing. Then relax the muscles and keep it relaxed for 10 seconds.

1. Arms: Tighten the fist on left side; release. Tighten the fist on right side; release. Feel the tension leave your body. Tighten your biceps by moving your forearms up toward your shoulders and making a traditional muscle. Hold, then relax. Tighten your triceps by holding out your arms in front of you and locking your elbows. Hold, then relax.

2. Head: Tense the muscles in your forehead by raising your eyebrows. Hold, then release. Then clench your eyelids shut. Hold, then relax. Imagine deep relaxation entering your face. Now, open your mouth as wide as you can, as you might when you're yawning, release.

3. Shoulders: Tense the muscles in your shoulders as you bring your shoulders up towards your ears. Hold, then relax.

4. Legs: Tighten your right thigh. Release. Then slowly, pull your toes towards you to stretch the lower leg and calf muscle. Repeat with the left thigh and left lower leg.

Caution: Use caution if you have a history of physical problems that may cause muscle pain and consult your doctor before you start.

Preparation: Choose surroundings that are naturally relaxing: your happy chair (not where you do bills), a designated area where you've journaled near a waterfall, or a fireplace area. Aromatherapy and music therapy can be helpful. The key is to minimize distractions--turning off the TV, turning off the radio, turning off the cellphone, allowing the urge to check email or text to subside. Let it go! The central key is to set aside the time and place for practicing relaxation skills.

HEALTHY NUTRITION

Your anxiety can affect your eating habits. Sometimes anxiety can lead a person to use eating as one of their tension reduction behaviors (TRBs). Consequently, this can lead to excessive eating and weight gain, resulting in health consequences such as heart disease, high cholesterol, diabetes, and obesity.

My colleague Dave Novicki, Ph.D. from the Michigan State Counseling Center who specializes in eating disorders and anxiety says: "Often, it is not about the eating, it is about the anxiety." Disordered eating can be a way that a person attempts to reduce their tension and anxiety. Whether disordered eating is a core issue, unhealthy eating usually involves eating sugars and sweets, salty foods (i.e. fries and potato chips), fats, and carbohydrates. Eating these "comfort foods" actually causes your anxiety to increase, because it disrupts healthy eating patterns. Poor nutrition also reduces the energy level that is required for anxiety management. In contrast, a healthy, balanced diet helps with anxiety reduction. There are so many strategies on healthy nutrition and dieting. It is easy to get sucked into some diet program.

> *Regularity in the hours of rising and retiring, perseverance in exercise, adaptation of dress to the variations of climate, simple and nutritious aliment, and temperance in all things are necessary branches of the regimen of health.*
>
> Lord Chesterfield

Dozens to hundreds of programs have been marketed in recent years. And, many of them have their own physicians providing expert testimony of the greatness of the program. The following are general guidelines for healthy nutrition planning based on traditional recommendations without gimmick diets or newer strategies.

PLENTY TO AVOID

One of the food items to eliminate for optimal health is *processed foods*: fast food from chains, boxed or frozen dinners, and even canned soups. Many turn to processed meats and processed cheese but these are to be avoided. *Trans fat* is an unsaturated fat with transisomer fatty acid. These lead to cardiovascular disease and are most notably found in fast foods, snack foods, fried food, and industrial baked goods.

Sugar is a drug, and we have become addicted to it. How many of us who eat semi-healthily will gladly indulge in the best ice cream. Sugar affects insulin levels which affects energy levels. Products to eliminate from your nutrition plan include soda pop, high fructose fruit juice, candy, cakes, and ketchup (which is loaded with sugar).

CAFFEINE IS A HUGE BARRIER FOR ANXIETY TREATMENT

One of the key barriers in anxiety treatment is heavy caffeine intake. Coffee and caffeinated teas should be eliminated or (before you throw this book away) decreased to one cup per day, if necessary. Caffeine can interfere with the absorption of important minerals like calcium or iron. In large quantities, it can lead to constipation and stomach problems. Caffeine abuse is highly problematic for individuals with anxiety. When I see individuals with basic anxiety and caffeine dependence, the solution often appears simple–eliminate the caffeine, get some exercise, regulate the sleep cycle, and talk about some of the problems.

OTHER EMPTY CALORIES AFFECT ENERGY LEVELS NEEDED FOR ANXIETY MANAGEMENT

Alcohol turns into sugar in your system and is very high in calories. Alcohol suppresses your emotions and puts a bandage on your problem. When consumed in excess, alcohol is physically dehydrating and draining on your body, leaving you fatigued. People who drink one night are less likely to exercise the next morning. When it comes to anxiety disorders, drinking to relieve anxiety is a trap. Clinicians should assess for all forms of substance abuse, particularly alcohol as strategies to relieve anxiety.

Other foods to avoid include *white flour*, which becomes sugar immediately in your body. It doesn't have much nutritional value, no fiber, and very few nutrients. White flour is a refined and processed food that takes away the minerals, nutrients, and fiber, which affects insulin levels making energy levels erratic. *Artificial colors* and *preservatives* are also to be avoided.

PLENTY TO EMBRACE: SUPER FOODS

There are plenty of foods that are rich in nutrients, phytochemicals, antioxidants, fiber, and essential fatty acids. Generally speaking, most people are aware of the importance of living a healthy life, consuming many servings of fruits and vegetables throughout the day. The foods are commonly called super foods because they contain a high nutrient and phytochemical density. Super foods often have fewer calories but significant amounts of nutrients that help prevent and, in some situations, reverse the well-known effects of aging, including cardiovascular disease, hypertension, particular forms of cancer, and Type II diabetes. Beyond prevention, consuming super foods increases energy, motivation, and good feelings.

The following are some of the essential super foods that are crucial for optimum health:

- Berries: Includes blueberries, blackberries, cranberries, raspberries, and strawberries. Contain fiber (pectin) and are high in nutrients and antioxidants.
- Extra Virgin Olive Oil: One ounce of oil contains 17.4 percent of the daily value for vitamin E. Several studies have demonstrated that adding olive oil to your regular diet could reduce your risk for breast and colon cancer, lower your blood pressure, and improve your cardiovascular system.
- Omega 3 Fatty Acids: Includes wild salmon, trout, sardines, and albacore tuna; these are great sources of omega-3 fatty acids.
- Green Tea: It's full of antioxidants.
- Whole Grains: Includes whole wheat, rye, barley, oats, quinoa and brown rice.

- Yogurt: This food promotes a healthy digestive system.

> The groundwork of all happiness is health.
>
> Leigh Hunt

- Cruciferous Vegetables: Includes broccoli, Brussels sprouts, cabbage, and cauliflower. These veggies contain many antioxidants and dietary fiber.

- Spinach: Contains calcium, magnesium, folate, fiber, and some omega-3 fatty acids. Research demonstrates an inverse relationship between spinach intake and cardiovascular disease, including stroke and coronary artery disease, and various cancers.

- Turkey: Highly nutritious and low in fat and one of the leanest meat proteins. It is rich in nutrients: niacin, selenium, vitamins B6 and B12, and zinc.

- Beans and Other Legumes: These foods contain protein, fiber, complex carbohydrates, and B vitamins.

> Food is your body's fuel. Without fuel, your body wants to shut down.
>
> Ken Hill

- Nuts and Seeds: Pecans, almonds, walnuts, flaxseeds, pumpkin seeds, and sunflower seeds contain protein and monounsaturated fatty acids which are good for the heart.

- Garlic: Has anti-inflammatory and antiviral properties and fights cancer and cardiovascular disease. It has many nutrients including allicin, a sulfur compound.

- Honey: Helps to inhibit the growth of bacteria, yeast, fungi, and viruses. Honey has significant levels of antioxidants.

Super foods are guaranteed to change your energy, health, and flavors in the kitchen. For more information on super foods, visit www.superfoodsrx.com.

THE POWER OF SAVORING

Taking time to eat and cook is sometimes called mindful eating. It usually involves immersing yourself in the eating experience. It starts with taking time to grocery shop rather than rushing through the store in haste (not always easy for parents with young kids).

> Let him who would enjoy a good future waste none of his present.
>
> Roger Babson

Mindfulness involves noticing the smells during the cooking. Eating involves taking each bite slowly, taking deep breaths between each bite, and taking time to notice the flavors and textures of each bite. Taking time to appreciate each moment is the essence of savoring every pleasurable experience slowly and delightfully. Savoring, being in the moment fully one with the food, is a great gift for freedom living.

Exercise: A Powerful Anxiety Antidote

A consistent exercise regimen can have a powerful effect on a variety of anxiety problems. Exercise helps you stay in shape physically, increase your vitality and energy, improve your self-esteem and self-confidence, and improve your appearance. Regular exercise helps bring healthy "release" or "relief" from that distress that builds up. In addition to regular and consistent sleep and a healthy super food diet, regular exercise makes a profound difference for living a life of freedom and happiness.

> *To enjoy the glow of good health, you must exercise.*
>
> Gene Tunney

There a variety of options to establish a program of exercise for yourself. For example, basketball on Monday nights, weight training on a couple of other days, mixed in with swimming and jogging. There are fabulous intense home fitness programs like P90X® and Insanity® that require high levels of motivation and passion. If you have tried these types of programs, Wow! But, there are many other types of activities that are all about living a healthy and balanced life style: Long-term running (including jogging), bicycling, hiking, dance classes, tennis, volleyball, soccer, Tai chi, yoga, karate classes, weight training, marathon running and various sports.

Name and Directly Confront the Excuse

One thing that this book is about is facing fears and anxieties head on as a way to get free. There are common excuses for avoiding exercise. Each one of these has a corresponding solution that is worth considering.

Excuse	Reframe
Avoid bodily sensations	You are ready to tolerate uncomfortable bodily sensations
I am unmotivated	Do it even if you don't feel like it.
I get fatigued	Exercise will improve your stamina
I can't fit it into my schedule	What are the ways I can make it a priority?

These are just a few of the simple ways to reframe these excuses. Usually, it involves taking a step back, gaining and broadening your perspective, and charging at life rather than away from it. Freedom from fears and anxiety is a life worth living.

References

Abramowitz, J.S. (1997). Effectiveness of psychological and pharmacological treatments for obsessive-compulsive disorder. *Joournal of Consulting and Clinical Psychology, 65*, 44-52.

American Psychiatric Association. (2013). *Diagnostic and statistical manual of mental disorders* (5th ed.). Arlington, VA: Author.

American Psychological Association (2005). Policy statement on evidence-based practice in psychology. Retrieved August 12, 2013 from: http://www.apa.org/practice/resources/evidence/evidence-based-statement.pdf

Ainsworth, M.D.S., & Bell, S.M. (1970). Attachment, exploration, and separation: Illustrated by the behavior of one-year-olds in a strange situation. *Child Development, 41*, 49-67.

Ainsworth, M.D.S., Blehar, M.C., Waters, E., & Wall, S. (1978). *Patterns of attachment: A psychological study of the strange situation.* Hillsdale, NJ: LawrenceErlbaum Associates.

Armita G., Selbing, I., Flygare, O., Öhman, A., & Olsson, A. (2013). Other people as means to a safe end: Vicarious extinction blocks the return of learned fear. *Psychological Science, 24*, 2135-2142.

Barlow, D.A. (2002). *Anxiety and its disorders:The Nature and treatment of anxiety and panic.* New York: Guilford Press.

Beck, A. T., Butler, A. C., Brown, G. K., Dahlsgaard, K. K., Beck, N., & Beck, J. S. (2001). Dysfunctional beliefs discriminate personality disorders. Behaviour Research and Therapy, *39*(10), 1213–1225.

Beck, A. T., Emery, G., & Greenberger, R. L. (1985). *Anxiety disorders and phobias: A cognitive perspective.* New York: Basic Books.

Beck, A. T. & Greenberg, R. L. (1988). Cognitive therapy of panic disorders. In R. E. Hales & A. J. Frances (Eds.), Review of psychiatry: Vol. 7 (pp. 571-583). Washington, DC: American Psychiatric Press.

Beck, A.T., Rush, A.J., Shaw, B.F., & Emery, G. (1979). *The cognitive therapy of depression.* New York: Guilford Press.

Bernstein, D. A. & Borkovec, T. D. (1973). *Progressive relaxation training: A manual for the helping profession.* Champaign, IL: Research Press.

Beutler, L.E., & Harwood, T.M. (2000). *Prescriptive psychotherapy: A practical guide to systematic treatment selection.* New York: Oxford University Press.

Binder, J. L., & Betan, E. J. (2013). Essential activities in a session of brief dynamic / interpersonal psychotherapy. *Psychotherapy, 50,* 3, 428-432.

Bisson, J.I.; Ehlers, A.; Matthews, R.; Pilling, S.; Richards, D.; Turner, S. (2007). "Psychological treatments for chronic post-traumatic stress disorder: Systematic review and meta-analysis". *The British Journal of Psychiatry 190,* 2, 97–104.

Bowlby, J. (1969). *Attachment and loss, Vol. 1.* New York: Basic Books.

Bremner, J. D., Elzinga, B., Schmahl, C., & Vermetten, E. (2008). Structural and functional plasticity of the human brain in posttraumatic stress disorder. *Progress in Brain Research, 167,* 171-186.

Breslau, N., Kessler, R.C., Chilcoat, H.D., Schultz, L.R., Davis, G.C., & Andreski, P. (1998). Trauma and posttraumatic stress disorder in the community: The 1996 Detroit Area Survey of Trauma. *American Journal of Psychiatry, 55,* 626-632.

Bretherton, I. and Munholland, K.A. (1999). Internal working models in attachment relationships: A construct revisited. In Cassidy, J. and Shaver, P.R. (Eds.) *Handbook of attachment: theory, research and clinical applications.* (pp. 89–111). New York: Guilford Press.

Buri, J. (2006). *How to love your wife.* Mustang, OK: Tate Publishing & Enterprises.

Burns, D.D. (1980). *Feeling good: The new mood therapy.* New York: Wm. Morrow and Co.

Casement, M.D. & Swanson, L.M. (2012). A meta-analysis of imagery rehearsal for post-trauma nightmares: Effects on nightmare frequency, sleep quality, and posttraumatic stress. *Clinical Psychology Review 32*(6): 566-574.

Cipriani, A., Hawton K., Stockton, S., Geddes, J.R. (2013). Lithium in the prevention of suicide in mood disorders: Updated systematic review and meta-analysis. *British Medical Journal, 346*, f3646.

Csikszentmihalyi, M. (1997). *Finding flow: The psychology of engagement with everyday life.* New York: Basic Books.

Davidson, J., Swartz, M., Storck, M., Krishnan R.R., & Hammet, E. (1985). A diagnostic and family study of posttraumatic stress disorder. *American Journal of Psychiatry, 142*, 90-93.

Dattilio, F.M. (2003). Emetic exposure and desensitization procedures in the reduction of nausea and a fear of emesis. *Clinical Case Studies, 2(3)*, 199-210.

Denker, P. (1946). Results of treatment of psychoneuroses by the G.P. *New York State Journal of Medicine, 46*, 2164-2166.

DeRubeis, R.J., Brotman, M.A., & Gibbons, C.J. (2005). A conceptual and methodological analysis of the nonspecifics argument. *Clinical Psychology: Science and Practice, 12*, 174-183.

Despland, J.-N., de Roten, Y., Despars, J., Stigler, M., & Perry, J. C. (2001). Contribution of patient defense mechanisms and therapist interventions to the development of early therapeutic alliance in a brief psychodynamic intervention. *Journal of Psychotherapy Practice & Research, 10*, 3, 155–164.

Duncan, B., Miller, S., & Wampold, B., & Hubble, M. (Eds.) (2010). *The heart and soul of change: Delivering what works in therapy* (2nd ed.). Washington DC: American Psychological Association.

Dunmore, E., Clark, D. M., & Ehlers, A. (2001). A prospective investigation of the role of cognitive factors in persistent posttraumatic stress disorder (PTSD) after physical or sexual assault. *Behaviour Research and Therapy, 39*, 1063–1084.

Easterbrook, J.A. (1959). The effect of emotion on cue utilization and the organization of behavior. *Psychological Review, 66*, 183-201.

Ekman, P. (1984). Expression and the nature of emotion. In K. Scherer and P. Ekman (Eds.), *Approaches to emotion* (pp. 319-343). Hillsdale, N.J.: Lawrence Erlbaum Associates.

Elliott, R., Bohart, A. C., Watson, J. C., & Greenberg, L. S. (2011). Empathy. *Psychotherapy, 48*, 43-49.

Ellis, A. (1962). *Reason and emotion in psychotherapy.* Seacaucus, NJ: Citadel Press.

Emmons, R.A., & McCullough, M.E. (2003). Counting blessings versus burdens: Experimental studies of gratitude and subjective well-being. *Journal of Personality and Social Psychology, 84,* 377-389.

Eysenck, H. J. (1952). The effects of psychotherapy: An evaluation. *Journal of Consulting Psychology, 16,* 319-324.

Eysenck, H. J. (1960). *Behavior therapy and the neuroses.* Oxford, U.K.: Pergamon Press.

Fluckiger, C., Del Re, A. C., Wampold, B. E., Symonds, D., & Horvath, A. O. (2012). How central is the alliance in psychotherapy? A multilevel longitudinal meta-analysis. *Journal of Counseling Psychology, 59,* 10-17.

Foa, E. B., Hembree, E. A., & Cahill, S. P. (2005). Randomized trial of prolonged exposure for posttraumatic stress disorder with and without cognitive restructuring: Outcome at academic and community clinics. *Journal of Consulting and Clinical Psychology, 73,* 953–964.

Foa, E. B., & Meadows, E. A. (1997). Psychosocial treatments for posttraumatic stress disorder: A critical review. *Annual Review of Psychology, 48,* 449-480.

Foa, E.B., & Kozak, M.J. (1996). Psychological treatments for obsessive-compulsive disorder. In: M.R. Mavissakalian 7 R.F. Prien (Eds.), *Long-term treatment of anxiety disorders* (*pp.*285-309). Wasington, D.C. American Psychiatric Press, Inc.

Frewen, P.A., Dozois, D.J.A., & Lanius, R.A. (2008). Neuroimaging studies of psychological interventions for mood and anxiety disorders: Empirical and methodological review. *Clinical Psychology Review, 28,* 228-246.

Gilbert, P., & Irons, C. (2005). Focused therapies and compassionate mind training for shame and self-attacking.In P. Gilbert (Ed.), *Compassion: Conceptualisations, research and use in psychotherapy* (pp. 263–325). London: Routledge.

Golkar, A., Selbing, I., Flygare, O., Öhman, A., & Olsson, A. (2013). Other People as means to a safe end: Vicarious extinction blocks the return of learned fear. *Psychological Science. 24*(11):2182-90.

Gould, R. A., Otto, M. W., & Pollack, M. H. (1995). A meta-analysis of treatment outcome for panic disorder. *Clinical Psychology Review, 15,* 819–844.

Gould, R.A., Otto, M.W., Pollack, M.H., & Yap, L. (1997). Cognitive behavioral and pharmacological treatment of generalized anxiety disorder: A preliminary meta-analysis. *Behavior Therapy, 28,* 285–305.

Hanrahan, F., Field, A.P., Jones, F.W. and Davey, G.C L (2013). A meta-analysis of cognitive therapy for worry in generalized anxiety disorder. *Clinical Psychology Review, 33*(1), 120-132.

Hariri, A., Drabant. E., Munoz, K., Kolachana, B., Mattay, V., Egan, M., et al (2005): A susceptibility gene for affective disorders and the response of the human amygdala. *Archives of General Psychiatry 62,* 146–152.

Hebb, D.O. (1949). *The organization of behavior.* New York: Wiley & Sons.

Hoehn-Saric, R., McLeod, D.R., Funderburk, F., & Kowalski, P. (2004). Somatic symptoms and physiological responses in generalized anxiety disorder and panic disorder. *Archives of General Psychology, 61,* 913-921.

Huppert, J.D. & Roth, D.A. (2003). Treating obsessive-compulsive disorder with exposure and response prevention. *Behavior Analyst Today, 4,* 59-63.

Institute of Medicine. (2001). *Crossing the quality chasm: A new health system for the 21st century.* Washington, D.C.: National Academy Press.

Jacobson, E. (1937). *Progressive relaxation.* (2nd ed.). Chicago, IL: University of Chicago Press.

Jobin J., Wrosch C., & Scheier M.F. (2013). Associations between dispositional optimism and diurnal cortisol in a community sample: When stress is perceived as higher than normal.*Health Psycholology* (epub ahead of print).

Landis, C. (1937). A statistical evaluation of psychotherapeutic methods. In L. E. Hinsie (Ed.), *Concepts and problems in psychotherapy.* New York: Columbia University Press.

LeDoux, J. E. (1996). *The emotional brain.* New York: Simon & Schuster.

Lesch, K. P., Bengel, D., Heils, A., Sabol, S. Z., Greenberg, B. D., Petri, S., et al. (1996). Association of anxiety-related traits with a polymorphism in the serotonin transporter gene regulatory region. *Science 274,* 1527–1531.

Luborsky, L., Singer, B., & Luborsky, L. (1976). Comparative studies of psychotherapies: Is it true that "everybody has won and all must have prizes"? In R.L. Spitzer & D.F. Klein (Eds.), *Evaluation of psychological therapies* (pp. 3-22). Baltimore: Johns Hopkins University Press.

Macklin, M.L., Metzger, L.J., Litz, B.T., McNally, R.J., Lasko, N.B., Orr, S.P., & Pitman, R.K. (1998). Lower precombat intelligence is a risk factor for posttraumatic stress disorder. *Journal of Consulting and Clinical Psychology, 66,* 323-326.

McNally, R. J., & Foa, E. B. (1987). Cognition and agoraphobia: Bias in the interpretation of threat. *Cognitive Therapy and Research, 11,* 567–581.

Mitte, K. (2005). A meta-analysis of the efficacy of psycho- and pharmacotherapy in panic disorder with and without agoraphobia. *Journal of Affective Disorders,* 88, 27–45.

McKay, D. & Moretz, M. W. (2008). Interoceptive cue exposure for depersonalization: A case series. *Cognitive and Behavioral Practice,* 15, 435–439.

Moylan, S., Giorlando, F., Nordfjærn, T., Berk, M. (2012). The role of alprazolam for the treatment of panic disorder in Australia. *The Australian and New Zealand Journal of Psychiatry, 46*(3), 212–224.

Nathan, P.E., & Gorman, J.M. (Eds.). (2007). *A guide to treatments that work.* (3rd Ed.) New York: Oxford University Press.

Norcross, J. C. & Lambert, M. J. (2011). Evidence-based therapy relationships. In J. C. Norcross (Ed.), *Psychotherapy relationships that work: evidence-based responsiveness* (pp. 3-21). New York: Oxford University Press.

Ophir, E., Nass, C., & Wagner, A.D. (2009). Cognitive control in media multitaskers. *Proceedings of the National Academy of Sciences of the U.S.A. 106*(37):15583-7.

Orlinsky, D. E.; Rønnestad, M. H.; Willutzki, U. (2004). Fifty years of psychotherapy process-outcomes research: Continuity and change. In M. J. Lambert, (Ed.). *Bergin and Garfield's Handbook of Psychotherapy and Behavior Change* (pp- 307-393). New York: Wiley.

Peterson, Christopher & Seligman, M.E.P. (2004). *Character Strengths and Virtues A Handbook and Classification.* Washington, D.C.: American Psychological Association Press and Oxford University Press.

Resnick, H.S., Yehuda, R., Pitman, R.K. and Foy, D.W. (1995) Effect of previous trauma on acute plasma cortisol level following rape. *American Journal of Psychiatry 152,* 1675-1677.

Rogers, C. (1957) The necessary and sufficient conditions of therapeutic personality change, *Journal of Consulting Psychology, 21*(2), 95-103.

Ross, L. (1977). "The intuitive psychologist and his shortcomings: Distortions in the attribution process". In Berkowitz, L. *Advances in experimental social psychology 10*. New York: Academic Press. pp. 173–220.

Rotter, J.B. (1954). *Social learning and clinical psychology*. New York: Prentice-Hall.

Roth, A., & Fonagy, P. (2005). *What works for whom? A critical review of psychotherapy research*. New York: The Guilford Press.

Schanche, E. (2013). The transdiagnostic phenomenon of self-criticism. *Psychotherapy, 48*, 3, 293-303.

Seligman, Martin E. P. (1991). *Learned Optimism: How to Change Your Mind and Your Life*. New York: Knopf.

Seligman, M.E.P. (1996). *The optimistic child: Proven program to safeguard children from depression & build lifelong resilience*. Boston: Houghton Mifflin.

Seligman, Martin E. P. (2002). *Authentic Happiness: Using the New Positive Psychology to Realize Your Potential for Lasting Fulfillment*. New York: Free Press.

Seligman, M.E.P. (2011). *Flourish*. New York: Simon & Schuster.

Sheehan, D.V., Sheehan, K.H., Raj, B.A. (2007). The speed of onset of action of Alprazolam-XR compared to Alprazolam-CT in panic disorder. *Psychopharmacology Bulletin, 40*(2): 63–81.

Siegal, D. & Hartzell, M. (2003). *Parenting from the inside out*. New York: Penguin Books.

Sloan, T., & Telch, M. J. (2002). The effects of safety-seeking behavior and guided threat reappraisal on fear reduction during exposure: An experimental investigation. *Behaviour Research and Therapy, 40*, 235–251.

Smith, M.L., & Glass, G.V. (1977). Meta-analysis of psychotherapy outcome studies. *American Psychologist, 32*, 752-760.

Spinazzola, J. Blaustein, M., & van der Kolk, B.A. (2005). Postrraumatic stress disorder treatment outcome research: The study of unrepresentative samples? *Journal of Traumatic Stress, 18*, 425-436.

Stewart, R.E., & Chambless, D.L. (2009). Cognitive-behavioral therapy for adult anxiety disorders in clinical practice: A meta-analysis of effectiveness studies. *Journal of Consulting and Clinical Psychology, 77*, 595-606.

Substance Abuse and Mental Health Services Administration, Office of Applied Statistics (2010). Drug Abuse Warning Network, 2007: *National estimates of drug-related emergency department visits. U.S. Department of Health and Human Services.* May 2010. Rockville. Available from: http://dawninfo.samhsa.gov/files/ed2007/dawn2k7ed.pdf

Swift J.K., & Derthick, A.O. (2013). Increasing hope by addressing clients' outcome expectations, *Psychotherapy, 50,* 284-287.

Szesko, P.R., Robinson, D., Alvir, J.M., Bilder, R.M., Lencz, T., Ashtari, M., et al. (1999). Orbital frontal and amygdala volume reductions in obsessive-compulsive disorder. *Archives of General Psychiatry, 56,* 913-919.

Task Force on Promotion and Dissemination of Psychological Procedures. (1995). Training in and dissemination of empirically-validated psychological treatments. *The Clinical Psychologist, 48*(1), 3-23.

Taylor S (1996) Meta-analysis of cognitive-behavioral treatments for social phobia. *Journal of Behavior Therapy and Experimental Psychiatry, 27,* 1–9.

True, W.R., Rise, J., Eisen, S.A., Heath, A.C., Goldberg, J., Lyons, M.J., & Nowak, J. (1993). A twin study of genetic and environmental contributions to liability for posttraumatic stress symptoms. *Archives of General Psychiatry, 50,* 257-264.

Tuckman, Bruce W. (1965) Developmental sequence in small groups, *Psychological Bulletin, 63,* 384-399.

U.S. Department of State Diplomacy in Action on Trafficking in Persons. http://www.state.gov/j/tip/

van Ingen, D., Freiheit, S., & Vye, C. (2009). From the lab to the clinic: A review of effectiveness studies of cognitive-behavioral treatments for anxiety disorders. *Professional Psychology: Research and Practice, 40,* 69-74.

van Ingen, D.J., & Novicki, D. (2009). An effectiveness study of group therapy for anxiety disorders. *International Journal of Group Psychotherapy, 59*(2), 243-251.

Whitaker, R. (2010b). *Anatomy of an epidemic; Magic bullets, psychiatric drugs, and the astonishing rise of mental illness in America.* New York: Crown Publishers.

Whiteside, S. P., Port, J. D., & Abramowitz, J. S. (2004). A review and meta-analysis of functional neuroimaging in obsessive-compulsive disorder. *Psychiatry Research: Neuroimaging, 132,* 69-79.

Appendix
Resources for Clinicians

THERAPIST RESOURCES

Abramowitz, J.S., McKay, D., & Taylor, S. (2008). *Obsessive-compulsive disorder: Subtypes and spectrum conditions.* New York: Elsevier.

Antony, M.M., Purdon, C., & Summerfeldt, L.J. (2007). *Psychological treatment of obsessive-compulsive disorder: Fundamentals and beyond.* Washington, DC: American Psychological Association.

Antony, M.M., & Rowa, K. (2008). *Social anxiety disorder: Psychological approaches to assessment and treatment.* Gottingen, Germany: Hogrefe.

Craske, M.G., Antony, M.M., & Barlow, D.J. (2006). Mastering your fears and phobias (2nd ed., therapist guide). New York: Oxford University Press.

Craske, M.G., & Barlow, D.H. (2007). *Mastery of your anxiety and panic* (4th ed., therapist guide). New York: Oxford University Press.

Foa, E.B., Hembree, E.A., & Rothbaum, B.O. (2007). *Prolonged exposure therapy for PTSD: Emotional processing of traumatic experiences* (Therapist guide). New York: Oxford University Press.

Hazlett-Stevens, H. (2008). *Psychological approaches to generalized anxiety disorder: A clinician's guide to assessment and treatment.* New York: Springer.

Hope, D.A., Heimberg, R.G., & Turk, C.L. (2006). *Managing social anxiety: A cognitive behavioral therapy approach* (Therapist guide). New York: Oxford University Press.

Resick, P.A., & Schnicke, M.K. (1996). *Cognitive processing therapy for rape victims: A treatment manual.* Newbury Park, CA: Sage Publications.

Recommended Self-Help Books to Supplement Therapy for Clients

Abel, J. L. (2010). *Active relaxation: How to increase productivity and achieve balance by decreasing stress and anxiety.* La Vergne, TN: Lightning Source.

Antony, M.M., & Swinson, R.P. (2008). *The shyness and social anxiety workbook: Proven, step-by-step techniques for overcoming your fear.* Oakland, CA: New Harbinger Press.

Burns, D.D. (1999). *The feeling good handbook.* New York: Plume Books.

Foa, E.B., & Wilson, R. (2001). *Stop obsessing! How to overcome your obsessions and compulsions.* New York: Bantam Books.

Jeffers, S. (2006). *Feel the fear and do it anyway.* New York: Ballantine Books.

Penzel, F. (2003). *The hair-pulling problem: A complete guide to trichotillomania.* New York: Oxford University Press.

Purdon, C., & Clark, D.A. (2005) *Overcoming obsessive thoughts: How to gain control of your OCD.* Oakland, CA: New Harbinger.

Wilhelm, S. (2006). *Feeling good about the way you look: A program for overcoming body image problems.* New York: Guilford Press.

Professional Resources

Clark, D. A., & Beck, A. T. (2010). *Cognitive therapy of anxiety disorders: Science and practice.* New York, NY: The Guilford Press.

McKay, D. & Storch, E. (Eds), (2011). *Handbook of anxiety disorders in children and adolescents.* Boston: Springer-Verlag.

Barlow, D. H. (Ed.) (2014), *Clinical handbook of psychological disorders: A step-by-step treatment manual* (5th ed.). New York, NY: The Guilford Press.

Associations

Association for Behavioral & Cognitive Therapies (ABCT) Website: www.abct.org. Includes professional membership and find a therapist

The American Academy of Cognitive and Behavioral Psychology (AACBP) Website: www.abpp.org. Includes: Find a board certified psychologist.

American Board of Professional Psychology Website: www.abpp.org

Academy of Cognitive Therapy (ACT) Website: www.academyofct.org. Includes: Find a therapist – low Cost cognitive therapist

WEBSITES

National Center for PTSD
www.ptsd.va.gov

National Institute of Mental Health
www.nimh.nih.gov

Daniel J. van Ingen's Anxiety & Trauma Practice Website
www.danvaningen.com

U.S. Department of Health and Human Services. Human Trafficking
www.acf.hhs.gov/trafficking/

U.S. Department of State Diplomacy in Action
Office to Monitor and Combat Trafficking in Persons
www.state.gov/j/tip

HEALTH AND WELLNESS WEBSITES AND APPS

Anxiety Coach. iPhone app. The Mayo Clinic.
Available at: https://itunes.apple.com/us/app/anxietycoach/id565943257?mt=8?
   View shared post

Ask the Dietician
www.dietician.com

The Superfoods
www.superfoodsrx.com

American Sleep Association
www.sleepassociation.org

1-800 Quit Now / stop smoking
www.smokingstopshere.com
Click calculators and converters, click health, and get cost of smoking calculator

Getting fit, losing weight, eating healthily
www.fitnessonline.com

For intense home fitness
www.beachbody.com